the humble little condom

AINE COLLIER

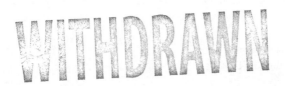
the humble little condom
A HISTORY

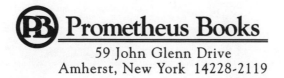

Prometheus Books
59 John Glenn Drive
Amherst, New York 14228-2119

Published 2007 by Prometheus Books

Inquiries should be addressed to

Prometheus Books
59 John Glenn Drive
Amherst, New York 14228–2119
VOICE: 716–691–0133, ext. 210
FAX: 716–691–0137
WWW.PROMETHEUSBOOKS.COM

11 10 09 08 07   5 4 3 2 1

Library of Congress Cataloging-in-Publication Data

Collier, Aine.
    The humble little condom : a history / by Aine Collier. — 1st American paperback ed.
        p. cm.
    Includes index.
    ISBN 978–1–59102–556–6
    1. Condoms—History. I. Title.

RC888.C65 2007
613.9'43509—dc22

2007027086

Printed in the United States of America on acid-free paper

contents

contents

acknowledgments

Eternal thanks to my dear friend and fellow historian Sharon Lee Olsen, California State University, Long Beach, for all of her efforts and scholarship and for thinking a history of the condom was a *good* idea; and to my beautiful daughters who stopped, after a few years, wrinkling their noses when it was mentioned.

introduction

An encourager of lewdness and lechery . . . impotent to deal with
   virile spermatozoon
A wonderful preventive against an accident which might lead to
   frightful repentance . . .

*B*audruche, *preservativo*, *gummi*, *peau divine*. By any other name, the little condom has a history that is anything but humble. Lauded and lionized for thousands of years, it has featured in the lives, loves, and letters of some of the most famous men in history: Shakespeare, Casanova, George Bernard Shaw, to name only a few. All appreciated the importance of using preventatives. But the story is about much more than who used them. It is a history of the human spirit, with all of its flaws and foibles.

While men—and women—have argued publicly over the morality of condom use throughout much of history, they have privately used them as both birth control and disease preventative. While the Church tried to dictate the dos and don'ts of the sex lives of its adherents, nuns and priests experimented with an interesting array of coverings. When women, immigrants, and Jews were unable to find work in mainstream business, they found a tidy and profitable niche making sheaths. By the late nineteenth century, rubber manufacture was big business, and by the early twentieth century, condoms had found their way onto Wall Street. Today it is a billion-dollar industry, dominated by some of the world's largest conglomerates.

The previously untold story of this little device is a study in human behavior, technology, disease, politics, psychology, and religion. It is funny, sad, sexist, sexy, and liberating. It is also a timely tale, as we live in an era when the world is dealing with the devastating effects of AIDS and, like the sexual plagues of the past, the only preventative remains *The Humble Little Condom.*

ONE

papyrus, serpents, and loincloths

THE ANCIENTS AND THE CONDOM

*L*ong before boy-pharaoh King Tut came to the throne, a prehistoric artist chronicled a man and a woman having sex—with his penis covered. The twelve-thousand-year-old cave art found in France's Grotte des Combarelles has no caption explaining just what the couple had in mind, but since their discovery in the late nineteenth century, archaeologists and historians have debated as to whether the "fecund" caveman and cavewoman were actually practicing safe sex.

Sexuality in ancient Egypt was open, untainted by guilt. Even the Egyptian gods were positively promiscuous, earthy enough to copulate with abandon, their lives filled with tales of adultery, incest, homosexuality, masturbation, and necrophilia. The Egyptians were sex obsessed and that obsession was often displayed in phallic worship: one of their creation stories has Chaos, their god of creation, masturbating, the act that produced all of the other gods in the Egyptian pantheon. Then there is the strange little god Bes, usually depicted as a dwarf who alternatively looked after childbirth and procreation—along with his other duties—and had a

---

WHAT DID THEY USE?
Crocodile dung mixed with honey and placed in the vagina of a woman prevents conception . . .
1850 BCE, a medical papyrus, written during the reign of Amenemhat III of the Twelfth Dynasty

---

phallus that reached all the way to the ground. Bes's importance grew to such an extreme that rooms where the inhabitants were most likely to have sex were dubbed "Bes chambers."

With all this love, and given the fact that Egyptians preferred small families, these technologically advanced people developed a number of methods to prevent too many or inconvenient pregnancies. Hieroglyphs from the second century CE recommended both male and female castration to prevent conception. Surgeries like the ovariotomy, the removal of the ovaries, were mentioned in medical papyri as a radical attempt to control fertility, but most methods were far less intrusive and were used only by women. Probably the most common was the *tampon*, a wadded-up linen strip, treated with spermicidal acidic oils or herbs. There were also herbal concoctions recommended in case the other precautions failed: recipes for drinks that would cause a woman to abort, a common practice that sparked no *moral* debates, were shared from generation to generation.

CHEWING GUM OR BIRTH CONTROL?
Pessaries, are "styptic, clogging, and cooling . . . cause the orifice of the uterus to shut before the time of coitus and do not let the seed pass into its fundus." In the second century CE, Soranus, noted Greek physician, acknowledged much of his knowledge of contraception came from the Egyptians. A favorite ingredient in Egyptian pessaries was acacia, a rubbery ingredient from the acacia tree. Egyptians also loved chewing gum, which was also made out of acacia gum (the real name for it!). Mixed with a little honey, this natural spermicide made a pretty tasty treat.

> ## ISRAELITES IN CAPTIVITY
> *During their time in Egypt, the Israelites learned about the pessary. Their version, called the "makk" or "mokh," was made with the standard Egyptian mixture of acacia and honey, but there is no evidence that they enjoyed chewing gum.*

Various medical papyri also describe devices and recipes for making *pessaries*, which are a sort of female condom that prevents semen from going all the way in, but does not actually *trap* it. Closer still to the male version, there was the halved, hollowed-out pomegranate shell, which served as a barrier. But what did the men use?

STRAP-ON PENISES, LOINCLOTHES, AND PAPYRUS

Their exact origins are unknown, but early penis sheaths undoubtedly developed out of the clothing styles favored by Egyptian men. Pharaohs and gentlemen of the upper ranks in Egyptian society wore short skirts, which were designed to project far out in front, emphasizing the wearer's anatomy with a triangular pleat, but it was the laboring classes who unintentionally designed the modern condom.

Worn for protection against sunburn, sand, and bug bites, working men's loincloths and girdles were little more than penis sacks, held on by a strip of cloth or a leather thong and tied around the waist. These were especially comfortable because they gave the workers freedom of movement as they fished, worked on their boats, and did laundry along the shore of the Nile. But by the Twelfth Dynasty (1350–1200 BCE) of the Middle Kingdom, there were written descriptions of men who were not common laborers wearing what were many years later dubbed *glans condoms*, small sheaths that covered only the top of the penis. These were made from oiled animal intestines or bladders, materials that remain popular even today. The fact that they were so small and made of such fine fabric meant they would not have been intended as a garment, or to be worn for an extended

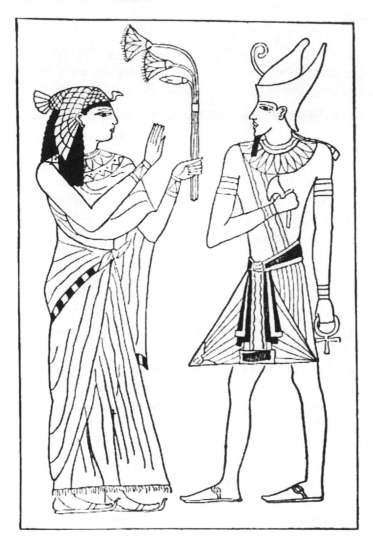

An ancient Egyptian "skirt"

period. The tiny bit of fabric would not have stood up to long-term wear and tear, sweat and sun, so even though the chronicler who described them did not come out and say just what the point of the diminutive garment was, the glans sheath would surely have been worn while having sex.

Even better examples are actual artifacts found in the tombs of aristocrats. These have yielded stashes of form-fitting penis sheaths made from soft animal skins and decorated with fur, some dyed in bright colors. Judging by what they packed, the men must have been deeply concerned about their sex lives in the Netherworld; along with their fancy condoms, they were also careful to include a supply of strap-on penises made from fine tortoise shell and mother of pearl. Some of these *tools* were carefully stored away for the journey, while others were already attached to the mummies.

HOW POPULAR WAS A PAPYRUS?

Ancient rumor has it that some pharaohs put on papyrus condoms before having sex with women they did not want to impregnate. Placing a paper condom (although these were made from only the most refined papyrus) over the royal member certainly illustrates the willingness of a powerful man to diminish his pleasure because of concern about sowing the royal seed in the wrong field. That has been a concern for many powerful men in history.

Perhaps it is odd that though they "designed" the first sheaths, there is no definitive evidence that the average Egyptian man thought of it as an actual birth control device.

Most likely only when a man of consequence was doubtful about his partner's "cleanliness" or was worried about leaving behind evidence of an adulterous relationship was he likely to seek protection. This remained a primary reason for men bothering with condomlike coverings for thousands of years. And of course, the blunting of sensation may also have been the culprit. Or perhaps because it was men who were the scribes of history, the papyri and other written discussions of contraception rarely did more than hint at men "taking responsibility."

ONE SPERM OR TWO? WHOSE FAULT IS IT ANYWAY?

As with other societies, early and modern, the ancient Greeks are a mixed bag when it comes to sex and sexuality. On the one hand, Greek art catalogs homosexual acts, naked men playing sports with other naked men, and all forms of prostitution. Rape was common, considered the right of men in a show of domination over women: the great god Zeus was the master rapist, disguising himself so that he could ravish both men and women.

Greek women had no choice about marriage partners and were considered property under law: they had little or no say over their own fates. Greek philosophers wrote of the ineptitude of women, and men generally thought all women suffered from penis envy.

Yet there is another, softer side to Greek society, some elements that lend a more sensual sense to what it was to be Greek. The Agora was a place in which people from all backgrounds came together and demonstrated the social and sociable side of daily life. And the Greek world was full of romantic gods and goddesses, bigger-than-life architectural wonders, and a passion for the word: drama, poetry, and comedy are reflective of the Greek spirit, of the people themselves.

In this potent, male-dominated, ugly-beautiful, sexually charged yet sexually ambivalent world, what was the common knowledge regarding contraception? And was the humble condom important?

> *A sign that the female does not emit the kind of seed that the male emits, and that generation is not due to the mixing of both as some hold, is that often the female conceives without experiencing the pleasure that occurs in intercourse.*
>
> Aristotle, fourth century BCE

In his book *Republic II* (372 BCE), Socrates described a pastoral paradise where there were only small families "lest they fall into poverty and war." He was concerned that too many mouths to feed could lead to hunger and despair. Hesiod also preached the small-family ethic, but his concern was about keeping the wealth in the family: "*Hope for an only son to nourish his father's house, for this is how wealth waxes in the hall.*"

Among the wealthy and middle classes, the Greek ideal was a boy to carry on the line and a girl to be married off to help create useful family alliances. Greek tradition required that sons inherit, and the always practical Greeks understood the potential damage to the wealth and power of the family if there were too many boys to provide for. But how did they engineer this "perfect" family?

Considering how long it took the modern Western world to scientifically prove just what causes pregnancy, it appears the ancients had some pretty good ideas as to what caused it and how to prevent it . . . and some interesting debates while figuring it all out.

Great thinkers like Plato and Aristotle argued that because of women's inferior status, it had to be men's semen that produced an embryo: "Woman in her conception and generation is but the imitation of the earth and not the earth of the woman." A woman's contribution to the process was her body as the receptacle for the man's seed.

But those who debated this singular theory were challenged by others who were not quite as antiwoman and definitely more logical. They put forth the argument that both men and women *had* to produce seed because children could look like either parent. Hippocrates was one of a number of medical philosophers who believed both parties produced semen and that conception was a very complex process involving both parents.

Whether they subscribed to Hippocrates' or Aristotle's theories, when physicians and philosophers wrote about birth control they made it clear that *that* was the woman's responsibility. There were many medical treatises noting recipes for contraceptive herbal concoctions, some to be taken internally, others made into pessaries: Aristotle wrote of witnessing the success of "anointing that part of the womb on which

HIPPOCRATIC CURES

Another abortificant . . . shake her under the armpits and give her to drink the petals. . . . Potent uterine abortificant . . . the roots of sweet earth almond.

From *Diseases of Women*,
a Hippocratic treatise

When a woman has intercourse, if she is not going to conceive, then it is her practice to expel the sperm produced by both partners whenever she wishes to do so.

Hippocrates in *The Sperm*,
fifth century BCE

the seed falls with oil of cedar, or with ointment of lead or with frankincense, commingled with olive oil." He even advocated for abortion (*phthorion*) should devices fail.

Aristotle was not alone: Hippocrates recommended that to end a pregnancy, a woman should jump up repeatedly, her heels touching her bottom. In a Hippocratic medical treatise, along with contraceptive advice (much of it bogus), there are a number of abortificants listed, some of them intended to be used as suppositories, others to be taken orally. And many of the methods advocated by Greek physicians, their recipes and directions, are so similar to the Egyptians' that it is obvious there was a lot of sharing going on across the Aegean.

SEMEN OF SERPENTS AND SCORPIONS

If life imitates art, then Greek legend is the best place to find evidence that the condom played a role in Greek life. In his second-century (CE) book of mythical tales *Metamorphoses*, Greek writer Antoninus Liberalis told the story of King Minos. The legend helps illuminate the use of condoms, but leaves the reader wondering just who wore them and why. Some translations of this mighty king's life have it that because of a curse put upon him by his wife—angry about his many infidelities—poor Minos had semen that contained serpents and scorpions. In order to prevent these monsters from killing his sex partners, Minos put on a condom, which captured the offending wildlife—an interesting spin on safe sex.

Other versions have it that it was Minos's partners who wore condoms. One way or the other, the legend tells us that these early people understood the significance of capturing a man's seed, but the origin of the Greek *sheath* is not quite so dramatic.

Like the Egyptians, Greek laborers wore brief coverings to protect them-

FEMALE CONDOMS

There are vague references in both Egyptian papyri and Greek texts to women wearing what can only be described as female condoms: but the writers indicate these were more "fashion" statements, making the wearers equals of men. This is strange but further proof of the odd place the condom had in early cultures.

CLEOPATRA

Probably because she had such all-consuming affairs with ancient Rome's most famous men, yet had only two children, it is assumed Cleopatra, Egypt's most famous and most infamous pharaoh, used a pessary as birth control. Since her lovers were also Roman soldiers, there is also the possibility that they used protection, too.

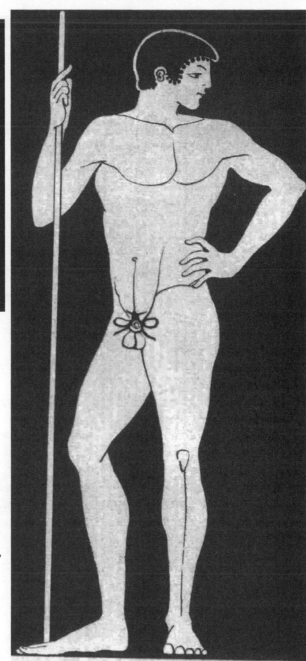

Kynodesme: "The dog knot"

19

selves from the elements while working outside and from possible damage while playing in sporting events. Evidence from a number of different dynastic periods has led some archaeologists to believe that there were at least two popular styles of sheaths used by the Greeks: they both bear a strong resemblance to the modern condom.

One of these was made up of a covering for the penis *and* a "testicle pouch." This double condom had a cord threaded through it that was tied around the wearer's waist. The other sheath was a single covering that did not cover the testicles and was held on by a ribbon. Some of these were quite elaborately dyed with vegetable pigments and were not always very form fitting. And some of them were really long—at least thirteen centimeters!

THE DOG KNOT

Controversial among those who have pondered the meaning of the condom in the lives of ancient Greeks is the kynodesme: literally "dog tie," or "dog knot." It was unlikely to have been related to the sex act, but does make for interesting speculation. When assembled, the dog knot resembled a condom, or sheath, but it was used by Greek athletes to confine their members during sporting events. It was a practical method for preventing the penis from flapping around during the games: a sort of ancient jockstrap.

A practice found later among African tribes, the dog knot is created by binding the end of the prepuce over the glans with a leather thong. The knot had to be untied in order to urinate and would have made having sex impossible. Knotting up the penis was also a symbol of athleticism among the naked athletes: according to Photius's Lexicon, it was a point of male sexual pride and supremacy for athletes to wear their penises all trussed up.

There are historians who believe the knot was also encouraged by trainers because it was thought that by tying the athletes up in knots, they would not be interested in sex; the Greeks believed that the sex act weakened men, which meant they were less likely to win.

PLEASE DON'T INTERUPTUS

But when did Greeks use condoms? In his discussion of family size, Plato talked of the "many devices available . . . to check propagation." Paros, seventh-century mercenary and poet, wrote, *"And, all her lovely body fondling, I also let go with my force, just touching, though her tawny down."* References like Paros's are peppered throughout Greek writing and have usually been interpreted to mean the practice of *coitus interuptus*, but there are those who believe these are subtle references to condom use.

In spite of the somewhat misogynistic—and sometimes confused—philosophers and medical men who dumped responsibility for small families on women, there were men who chose to practice birth control on their own. Herodotus reported that Pisistratus, the sixth-century tyrant of Athens, "did not want to have children by his new wife and so had intercourse with her not according to custom." Again, experts have interpreted this as coitus interuptus, or anal intercourse, but it is very possible that Pisistratus was actually doing what the Egyptian pharaohs had done. He may have used one of those animal intestine condoms to make sure he remained the sole power in Athens.

In a society as sexually charged as that of the Greeks, where concubinage, homosexuality, and elaborate orgies were an accepted part of life, it seems likely that the condom, however surreptitiously, was a quiet addition to the more public birth control methods favored by the Greeks (especially by those men who trusted no one but themselves to prevent an unwanted pregnancy, or chose to explore sex with women of the lower ranks or slaves). In a society that was so promiscuous, it simply made sense. If it was good enough for a Greek king, it was surely good enough for the rest of Greek society.

ANCIENT GREEK MARRIAGE TOAST
May my enemies fall in love with women and my friends with boys.

CONTAGION, CONFUSION, AND ROMAN SEX

I hate and I love. Perhaps you ask why I do that?
Catullus (second century CE)

When Rome consumed the older and more sophisticated world of the Greeks, Romans inherited a great deal of information about how to prevent unwanted pregnancies and avoid sexually transmitted infections. And, like the Greeks, men called all the shots. Sex in ancient Rome was decidedly one sided: men could get it anytime, anywhere. Exotic sex was easy to find; orgies and group sex were common, as were homosexual encounters. Household slaves and prostitutes provided a handy outlet for bored husbands.

On the other hand, women's role in Roman society was completely scripted: wealthy girls were married to cement family alliances, and poor girls fended for themselves. Sex and love were not synonymous, and sex outside of marriage (for women) was a no-no. Cato's examination of how husbands and wives were treated under law illustrates the differences between the consequences for men versus women if caught committing adultery: *"If you take your wife in adultery you may freely kill her without a trial. But if you commit adultery, or if another commits adultery with you, she has no right to raise a finger against you."* Men dictated the laws and they benefited from their own handiwork.

Though much has been made by historians of the importance of family and children to the Romans, it was not a Roman goal to keep wives barefoot and pregnant. They wanted small families. Reminiscent of the Greeks, the ideal was to have no more than one or two children in order to prevent the splitting up of family wealth as a result of too many boys to provide for and too many girls—often married off by twelve—who were worthless except to create or maintain family alliances.

But there was another reason, one a number of increasingly worried emperors tried to address, but with no luck: big families cost a lot to rear, and wealthy and middle-class women did not appreciate the wear and tear on their bodies. Some well-to-do Romans were even honest enough to say that they did not want a lot of children because it would prevent them from enjoying the many entertainments available in Roman cities, cutting into their time at the Coliseum. But their commitment to small families was not a minor footnote in the history of the Roman Empire. It was a contributing factor to its fall.

Because the small-family philosophy was so widespread, by the first century CE the population of free Roman citizens had plummeted, making it difficult to fill the ranks of the huge army and to provide the infrastructure necessary to maintain history's largest empire. In fact, Augustus was so worried about the common practice of "family limitation" that he demanded the Senate pass legislation making any kind of contraception illegal. Roman literature, however, makes it clear that in spite of the heavy penalty for breaking this law, Romans remained dedicated to small-family size.

> *For a woman forbids herself to conceive and fights against it.*
> Lucretius, 50 BCE

Pater familias, father of the family, is a term that refers to Roman men's complete and legally sanctioned control over the family, including wives. A woman could say nothing about the dalliances between her husband and a pretty slave girl: a wife had little influence in her own home. In spite of that low standing, or possibly because of it, Roman men, like their Greek counterparts, expected their wives to deal with contraception. Though a serious burden, this responsibility may actually have empowered some women and allowed them to have the final say in the number of children they had, or even to stray from the constraints of dominant husbands and a demanding code of law.

Although plenty of fairly common Roman contraceptives were no more than magical potions—a squashed spider worn under the left arm was a favorite—Roman women also had very potent birth control choices at their disposal. Herbal potions from commonly available plants like Queen Anne's lace were effective contraceptives, and tampons soaked in oils or acidic liquids—identical to those used by Egyptian women—were very popular. But did Roman men participate in family planning?

The Romans believed that semen was the essence of a man's "maleness." They were very public about worship of the *fascinum*—phallus—which was the symbol of both war and love. Roman bakers were proud of their perfect loaves of phallus-shaped bread. Covering the coveted object might seem anathema to these penis-lovers, but there are many veiled references to men covering themselves with condomlike sheaths. The clues to Roman condom use can be found in the creative language of reticent Roman chroniclers and in hints peppered throughout Roman literature: medical, military, fictional, and personal.

Whether from concerns about being caught in adulterous affairs with the wives of important men, from the fear of infection, or from the commitment to assure a small family, even in this male-dominated society, Roman men did use protection.

BOY THAT STINGS!

> *Gossip records a miracle: that to rub it all over the male part before coition prevents conception.*
>
> Pliny the Elder, first century CE

Although most of the devices and concoctions recommended to Roman men for protective or preventative use while having sex were at best quirky, they do offer a glimpse at how serious Roman men were about avoiding the unfortunate consequences of having sex, especially illicit sex.

Pliny the Elder's miracle involved rubbing the penis with cedar oil, which may have stung a bit, but Pliny's was not the only unguent recommended as a penis protector or covering. There were plenty of recipes directing men to brew up thick, gooey substances to apply to the penis before sex. The sometimes greasy, often smelly concoctions could not "catch the seed," but their astringent and highly acidic ingredients had spermicidal qualities that may or may not have been effective.

THE CONDOM CIRCUS AND FILTHY SLIPPERS

Although those gooey coverings were examples of men participating in birth control, when it came to condoms, like those who came before and who would follow, it was all about protecting the men from the women. A

PROSTITUTED EUPHEMISMS: LATINATE TERMS FOR *PROSTITUTE*

spurcae lupae—filthy whore

meretrix—harlot, the classiest member of the profession

prostibula—one who sits in front of her stall, waiting for customers

proseda—she who stands in front of her stall

nonariae—she who is forbidden to appear before the ninth hour (no afternoon delights)

mimae—mime players, who were always assumed to be (and usually were) prostitutes

cymbalistriae—cymbal players (strange intersection)

ambubiae—singing girls, same

citharistriae—harpists, same

scortum—strumpet who meets customers in secret

scorta erratica—streetwalkers who were quiet about their profession

busturiae—prostitutes who hung out around tombs and at funerals (what a way to find a customer)

copae—barmaids

delicatae—mistresses

famosae—soiled doves (women from good families who became professionals)

dois—whores who were naked and beautiful

lupae—she wolves, either because of the sounds they made while having sex or because they were animal-like in their lusts

aelicariae—baker's girls

noctiluae—nightwalkers

blitidae—also the name of a cheap drink sold in the crummy taverns in which these women plied their trade

forariae—country girls who hailed travelers along roadsides

gallinae—"hens who scatter everywhere," these were thieving prostitutes who stole from their clients

amasiae—vamps, these girls were devoted to the worship of Venus

rare exception was after a day at the games.

The deadly tournaments fought by brave gladiators in the Roman amphitheaters were known for more than their bloodletting. They were also notorious for their after-the-show trysts. It was a dirty little secret that married women found the winning gladiators very, very sexy—the more battle-worn and scarred, the better. Well-to-do women watched enthralled as their men fought, then they met up with their tough paramours after the show. Although adultery was common, it was still dangerous for the woman, legally punishable by death. That and the fact that the women did not want to

> ## ROMAN MISOGYNY
>
> *Citizens, if it were possible to go entirely without wives, as would deliver ourselves at once from this evil; but the laws of nature have so ordered it that we can neither live happy with them nor continue the species without them, we ought to have more regard for our lasting security than for our transient pleasures.*
> Censor Q. Metellus Macedonicus, 131 BCE, on the concerns over the shrinking population of Rome
>
> *Males have figured out all the back alleyways of sex, crimes against nature; but women figured out abortions.*
> Pliny the Elder, first century CE

spoil it all by becoming pregnant made contraception vital, but it was not the only consideration for these daring women: gladiators were not the cleanest choice of lovers. It has been posited that part of the lusty bargain was the promise to use sheaths to protect the ladies from infection and detection. And then there were the other "ladies."

Roman prostitutes were referred to as the *publica via*, the public footpath, inferring the prostitute's role in society as analogous to all that was dirty and degrading. *Spurcae*, dirt, was used in some of the most common metaphors describing prostitutes. Yet the great Roman writers speak often of the necessity of prostitution in Roman society, as an outlet for men who did not want to impregnate their wives, who were away from home a great deal traversing the empire, or who wanted to explore the kinkier side of life.

Prostitution was so prevalent and varied in ancient Rome that there were dozens of Latinate euphemisms describing prostitutes and their wares. Latin was so deeply influenced by the Roman love-hate relationship with prostitutes, even architectural terms were borrowed to describe paid-for sex. Streetwalkers—those who were not managed by pimps or who did not operate out of brothels—used the arcades, the corridors formed by the large arches at circus buildings common throughout Roman cities and towns, to turn quick tricks. These little hideaways, or fornices, provide the root for the modern English word fornication.

Prostitutes' vital, and reviled, role in society is even reflected in Augustine's writing: "Banish prostitutes from society and you reduce society to chaos through unsatisfied lust." His statement illustrates the Roman ambiguity over prostitution, at once a necessity *and* a degrading, vilified practice.

Indeed, the most insulting dirty reference about the Roman prostitute and her clients is the *filthy slipper*, a dual comment on her cleanliness and the use of condoms. The men who used the services of prostitutes, especially those men with power and place in society, did not want to suffer the all-too-possible contagion when "walking the public footpath"; they wore filthy slippers for protection.

NEIGH-WINNIE AND THE MAGIC CONDOM

One of the many odd Roman condoms was also purported to have had magical qualities that protected the users from pregnancy and evil spirits. Magic or not, it was definitely unique not only for being a joint effort but also because of the material it was fashioned from. To make the *magic condom*, the woman was directed to collect a large handful of fur from a she-mule's mane. As a sort of foreplay, the man and the woman hand-wove a *furry condom* and then she helped him put it on.

The origins of this she-mule-hair condom have been lost to time, but it leaves the modern reader wondering which would be the greatest obstacle to enjoyment and safety: the possible leakage or the incredible itch. Maybe that was the magic . . . managing to have sex wearing the strange contraption.

MOUNT VESUVIUS'S RASH
AND FLEXING THEIR MUSCLES

Although there are many veiled references to condom use by Roman men, they were most commonly used by one group: Roman soldiers. During many campaigns, the armies of Rome were supplied with comfort women, usually captives taken after battle. These poor women made up the majority of workers in the military brothels, but there were also women who voluntarily followed the army, living with and around the soldiers, accompanying them from campaign to campaign. At the 106 BCE Battle of Arousio (yes, really), for example, there were eighty thousand troops and forty thousand *camp followers.*

Camp followers at any battle or post were a mixed group; some were the legal wives of soldiers who dragged their household goods and children along with them, but more commonly, they were prostitutes who found the army a steady means of employment. Although there was a certain reciprocity in the lifestyle, sex for security, the casual nature of these relationships had its risks.

AH, THE JOYS OF BEING A WOMAN!

Permissiveness towards women is harmful to the purposes of the community and to the happiness of the state . . . for they live without restraint in every kind of indulgence and luxury.

Aristotle, *Politics*, 1296 BCE

Women! This coin which men find counterfeit!
Why, why, Lord Zeus, did you put them in the world,
in the light of the sun? If you were so determined
to breed the race of man, the source of it
should not have been women. Men might have dedicated
in your own temple images of gold,
silvers, or weight of bronze, and hues have bought
the seed of progeny, . . . to each been given his worth in sons
according to the assessment of his gift's value. So we might
have lived in houses free of the taint of women's presence.

Euripides, fifth century BCE

Prior to the fifteenth century, it is not known if sexually transmitted diseases were a serious public health threat. Certainly sexually transmitted infections were known and dreaded, hence wealthy men protected themselves when they used the services of prostitutes. Reports like the one from Aretaeus the Cappodocian (second century CE) might have been describing a mild precursor to gonorrhea or more likely something like a yeast infection when he spoke of men with "not,

SURE-FIRE CURES

In Corinth, clay models of a man's genitals were considered a reliable cure for healing sexually transmitted infections; there is no record as to how the models were "applied," but they are believed to have been prescribed to women by priests connected to the cult of Asclepius, God of healing.

indeed, a deadly affection, but one that is disagreeable and disgusting even to hear of." Aretaeus blames women for the problem: "Women also have this disease, but their semen is discharged with titillation of the parts, and with pleasure, and from immodest desires of connection with men. But men have not the same prurient feelings."

Who carried which kind of infection was not as important to the common foot soldier, however, as it was to the medical minds of the time. What many military men did know and care about was that having sex meant exposure to a variety of nasty infections. Legend has it Roman soldiers lumped these together with the term *Mount Vesuvius's rash*.

Roman legions often kept herds of goats with them, as a hardy and handy source of meat and milk. Savvy soldiers (like those before and after) figured out what to do with the otherwise-useless goat bladders, or intestines, which made pretty fair penis sheaths. This could easily have been a technique inherited when they invaded the Greeks. The soldiers covered their glans using pieces of dried and stretched bladder and kept the condoms in place by tying small pieces of leather or string around the top of the penis.

In Roman Britain, officials whose job it was to oversee the business of skins and hides were directed to supply preprepared skins to armies going off to war—an important military lesson learned and unlearned by later armies from the seventeenth to the twentieth centuries.

HELMET OR CONDOM? THE ROMAN CODPIECE

One of the earliest condomlike devices mentioned by a Roman chronicler was intended to be used only by thespians. Meant more or less for birth control, it was a cross between a condom and a helmet. Metal was hammered and shaped to look like a bowler hat, which fit directly over the glans. The device was attached by thongs strung through holes in the helmet, then tied around the waist—a sort of Roman codpiece. This metal condom was the brainchild of theater owners and managers, who worried constantly about their male actors' and singers' sexual indiscretions with wealthy patronesses.

In spite of the fact that entertaining was considered a demeaning profession, fit only for men of the lower classes, and women were not allowed on the stage, there were plenty of married women in the audience. The theater managers were concerned that the more handsome and talented actors would pursue or be pursued by the women they were entertaining, distracting the actors and causing potential legal problems for the theater owners when angry husbands found out. The most popular entertainers were the mimes, who were so successful at their portrayal of sex that lots of women wanted to participate.

The penis-helmet ensured there was no "display" under scant costumes or loose robes, but the real purpose was to make the actors uncomfortable in their hard, cold "container."

It does not appear though to have had much affect on inhibiting the entertainers' libidos and keeping their minds on the job; or distracting the women. Roman chroniclers like Juvenal (first century CE) wrote with disgust about actors, calling them base "prostitutes." He saved his sharpest criticisms, however, for the rich women who found actors extremely attractive: "As she watches the pantomime Bathyllus (an actor) playing the role of Leda . . . all at once Apula (a wealthy spectator) moans in drawn-out ecstasy, as if in a man's embrace."

The most exotic male covering in the history of the Roman Empire, maybe in all of Western history, was also the brainchild of the Roman soldier. Legends about just how far victorious Roman soldiers would go to prove—or celebrate—their superiority in the field tell of a remarkable covering. This *victory condom* was made out of the muscle (some versions say just the skin) from an enemy soldier defeated in battle. From the sinewy material, the Roman soldier fashioned his covering by stretching the muscle tissue and soaking it in oil to soften it. Whether the material was shaped in place then attached with a ribbon or string is unclear, but the victory condom was a symbol of the warrior's bravery and skill in battle . . . and with women. It is only a guess that the women who were at the receiving end of this device may have had mixed feelings about its use.

DID THE CONDOM FALL, TOO?

When the Roman Empire fell, and the Western half of that once great power was left to fend for itself, the rich world of science and politics the Romans had borrowed, created, and spread throughout their world shrank, taking almost a millennia to fully reawaken. But does that mean that those left to cope with the fractured remnants of empire lost the knowledge of the ancients? Was there a *feudal condom*?

TWO

from sex for "delit" to the great pox

LOVE IN EARLY MODERN EUROPE

A husband would please me though
But to bear children I believe is a great penance
Since the breasts fall down and the belly becomes heavy and
*   burdening.*

By a thirteenth-century poetess

uried deep in the ancient art, poetry, and chronicles of the Egyptians, Greeks, and Romans is the story of the ancient sheaths that men wore mostly to protect themselves from disease and sometimes from the entanglements of an unwanted pregnancy. But for some reason, traditional historians of the Middle Ages have insisted that when Rome fell, the understanding and practice of any sort of birth control was lost, and that the medievals did nothing to limit family size; and of course they lived short, brutish, and sexually ambivalent lives, so there was no need.

Not quite.

Although there were cataclysmic changes that accompanied the end of empire, and the center of power was lost to that localized notion of rule called feudalism, by the eleventh century medieval treatises, diaries, and literary sources were full of references (some veiled, many literal) to and about human sexuality, including directions on how to prevent or end pregnancy.

And they more than hint at the fact that the condom did have a quiet role in the lives of some early Europeans. In fact, in many ways this unique period in Western history could be interpreted as a pretty sexy one; by the 1000s, popular literature portrayed the emergence of serious sexual exploration, with men and women as both romantic partners and combatants in the medieval version of the *battle of the sexes*. At the same time, the Church was becoming very concerned about dictating the terms in regard to what went on behind closed doors. However, as so often happens in history, what was preached was not always what was practiced—the Church provided a cozy niche for those who enjoyed lots of sexual experimentation and exploitation: some friars, nuns, and even a pope or two were anything but chaste.

OUTLAWING *DEVIZES*

The legal codes of England's Edward I provide a serious glimpse into how widespread the practice of birth control was in the early Middle Ages; his laws made it illegal to provide a woman with any kind of birth control *devize* or advice. And like the Roman emperors who tried to outlaw the practice, codes of law could do little to prevent it: female neighbors, friends, and relatives quietly educated one another, and there were even those who actually made a living from growing the herbs and collecting the flora necessary to make contraceptive mendicants. As history proved—then and later—watchful leaders were rarely successful in catching and prosecuting wrongdoers because as long as people wanted to "check propagation" so badly that they would thumb their noses at the law—and others found the practice profitable enough to make crossing the legal line worthwhile—there would be no way to prevent it. Perhaps even more telling is that there was nothing mentioned in Edward's codes about punishments for men if they got caught informing about or selling *devizes*.

> *Si non caste tamen caute. . . . If not chastely at least cautiously, with care, with precautions.*
>
> A common "philosophy" about sex,
> eleventh through thirteenth centuries

In his *Summa conservationis et curationis*, thirteenth-century Italian physician William of Saliceto included a chapter on how to prevent pregnancy with mostly herbal mixes; he also explained how to induce abortion. His methods were borrowed from the more advanced medical knowledge of the Arab world, which in turn took a great deal from the ancients, but it was not the academics or the physicians of the Middle Ages who were the movers and shakers in the world of birth control. The very best source of information about just what the medievals *knew* was the clergy.

Throughout the Middle Ages the Church got more and more involved in people's daily lives, especially regarding sexual relations. Clergymen pushed for doctrines that dictated sex was meant only for the marriage bed and strictly for the purposes of reproduction—enjoyment was out. Church policy discouraged the faithful, as it still does, from practicing "abortion or contraception."

This very public campaign to limit people's libidos makes the fact that it was the Church that housed most of the information about medieval birth control truly ironic. Even more amazing is that it was churchmen who performed much of the research that advanced the understanding of reproduction—and how to prevent it.

Some of the information came from surviving Greek and Roman treatises, painstakingly copied in Latin by patient monks hidden away in their scriptoriums. But monks did more than just copy old recipes. They actually experimented with the contraceptive concoctions and decoctions them-

USEFUL AND USELESS PREVENTATIVES

Tisanes of lavender, parsley, and marjoram were considered potent contraceptives by practitioners of German folk medicine. Teas brewed from the seeds of fruitless trees were thought to have contraceptive qualities—after all, if the tree was fruitless, it made sense the woman who drank the tea would be, too. Some of these worked, some did not. Willow bark tea was also thought not only to act as a contraceptive, but would actually cause women to become sterile. Seeds from wild flowers like Queen Anne's lace—which really is a potent contraceptive—were also popular oral contraceptives. Men were not completely left out: "Camphor through the nostrils by its odor castrates men." Interesting, but incorrect—camphor is actually a natural aphrodisiac.

selves. Growing, harvesting, mixing, and cooking the wide variety of flowers, herbs, and wild flora was a daily obsession for a cadre of padres. How they knew their brews worked is more difficult to ascertain, but many of the potions contained ingredients modern science has proven effective.

Conversely, well-traveled and worldly men—and women—of the Church actually wrote about contraception in their diaries and letters, some of which became books of wisdom shared throughout their own dioceses and beyond. These mostly fourteenth-century Mendicant and Dominican friars learned a great deal in the confessional. When the brothers and priests heard the confessed sins of their parishioners, specifically those who felt a little bit guilty about making sure they did not become pregnant, infected, or did not "plant a seed" in the wrong furrow—and how they engineered it—the churchmen had a pretty good idea of just what worked and just how many people were actively trying to avoid unfortunate accidents. They also knew who was sleeping with whom.

English friars like John Bromyard of Hereford and William of Pagula from the Salisbury diocese, along with French, Portuguese, and Italian brothers, peppered their written treatises with statements like: "ne impraegnaretar"—*lest she become pregnant*; "ne habeat plures filios"—*in order not to have more children*; "propter quod impediatur concepcio partus"—*whereby conception be prevented*. The references to pregnancy and prevention were all part of the clergymen's practical advice, intended, of course, for married parishioners, passing on what the good friars had learned from those same folks.

THE TURIN PAPYRUS
The sexiest papyrus found to date has to be the Turin, written during the time of the New Kingdom. It features every kind of sexual indulgence. With men pleasing men, men with enormous erections, and nude young women with much older men, it is a great example of antique pornography.

A fourteenth-century English Carmelite nun went even further when she argued that birth control was a way to distinguish "man from beast . . . but man does not just aim at generating offspring [for] the multiplication of the Species, like a beast; he aims at living a good and peaceful life with his wife." She did not give any advice as to how to limit offspring, but she provided a glimpse into the beginning of the birth control wars as they would be fought within the Church itself.

On the flip side, though she was against the practice of any kind of birth control, Saint Catherine of Sienna was not shy about discussing it in public. She bemoaned the fact that contraception was the most frequent sin of "the married" who did not have as much "conscience" about it as their "other sins," like stealing, swearing, and gluttony.

And then there was Pierre Clergue of Montaillou, often referred to as the thirteenth century's "fornicating priest," who noted in his diaries that he made sure his lover was using what sounded like a female condom when he asked if she was using "their method" of birth control.

THE POMEGRANATE IS BACK

Although not a member of the Church, thirteenth-century Italy's Dame Torotula, called history's first woman gynecologist, also offered rather vague advice to women with "female troubles." She recommended that old favorite the pomegranate be worn as a pessary. Just as in ancient Egypt, women were told to cut the fruit in half, hollow it out, and insert it. She left out when and why a woman should wear a pomegranate, but considering the parallels between the old world and the emerging modern one, the dame was probably just being cautious (or coy) when she committed a bit of her contraceptive knowledge to vellum, trying to pass on her wisdom without setting herself up for prosecution by overzealous authorities.

PERSIAN PROTECTION

Again, thanks to Church documents, there is plenty of evidence that men did practice birth control. What is missing is any mention of preventatives against sexually transmitted infection,

JESUS AND FAMILY PLANNING
Though he did not speak specifically about birth control, Jesus of Nazareth was a proponent of one-child families.

DE COITUS LIBER

In his treatise On Sexual Intercourse, *eleventh-century Constantine the African, another busy monk who while cloistered in the Benedictine abbey at Monte Cassino translated preexisting Arabic text into Latin, wrote about some interesting—and somewhat confusing—methods of birth control. Among other things, Constantine advised using the rinds of melons and gourds. These, he assured his readers, work well in lessening a man's libido, but he seems to be referring to using them as a receptacle, since he also says that if the hollowed-out shells are used "correctly," then they are good at "drying out the semen." Although he is terribly vague, it seems that he may be referring to something akin to the ancient Japanese use of tortoiseshell condoms.*

In the Avicenna, *another Latin translation of a famous Arabic medical text (the* Ibn Sina*), the Latin translator, for whatever reason, left out a condom recipe found in the original Arabic. The Arabic version recommended that a "liquid condom" be made out of white lead. Directions on how to wear the lead condom were not included.*

the most common reason for men of the ancient world's willingness to cover up. By the Middle Ages, however, the understanding of the relationship between sex and infection was only tacitly acknowledged. The Norman English referred to *la chaude pisse* (hot piss), a common ailment thought to have been caused by having sex with a dirty prostitute. By the twelfth century there was a law that prohibited brothel keepers of Southward in London from allowing "women suffering from the perilous infirmity of burning" to work for them; and fourteenth-century English references to a similar problem included the *gleet*, *droeppert*, and *tripper*. But until the late Renaissance, these infections (which, as with earlier periods, some medical historians believe were mild forms of gonorrhea) were all lumped together along with diseases unrelated to sex, specifically leprosy. However, during the Middle Ages, the coverings used by men were not intended as protection from disease. They were birth control.

As demonstrated by William of Saliceto's work, there is evidence that the earliest trailblazers who reestablished contact with the new Islamic world returned from their travels with information about contraceptive methods, which included the condom. Persians, for instance, mention penis coverings made from leathery materials made to be worn while having sex; this rein-troduced or reinforced the use of the quiet experimentation with the condom in Europe.

Often called the "Hippocrates of the Islamic world," Abu Bakr Muhammed ibn Zakariya al-Razi (900 CE) was a Persian doctor who wrote about contraception. His work was as much an exploration of moral dos and don'ts as a contraception "how to," but buried in his philosophies al-Razi listed the reasons why there were times when semen should not be allowed "in." Like his Roman and European counterparts, al-Razi's wording is typi-cally vague, but his explanation of how to avoid getting it "in" while still having sex sounds a lot like using a condom. Others in the Islamic world sug-gested condomlike coverings made from tar, which could not have been much worse than the male birth control recommended by a twelfth-century Jewish physician: "Soak the penis in the pure juice of the onion."

COURTLY OR CORPOREAL?

> *And there go the fair and courteous ladies, who have friends—two or three—besides their wedded lord.*
>
> Twelfth-century verse

Literature of the Middle Ages celebrated courtly love, traditionally defined as a chaste and pure relationship between the brave knights and lovely ladies of the European courts. The men worshiped and adored their beloveds from afar, their love remaining unrequited. But medieval poetry and less romantic tales recount some satisfyingly sexy relationships.

> *Here youths and their lemans [mistresses]*
> *Stroll through leafy groves where*
> *Grass sprung up as thicke set*
> *And soft as any velvet*
> *On which men might their lemans lay*
> *As on a featherbed to play.*
>
> Chaucer, *Book of Duchess*

In other works, Chaucer was not quite so subtle when he referred to the relationships of court members; he also *proved* that medievals did enjoy sex—and practiced birth control (both of which he disapproved). In the *Nun's Priest's Tale*, courtly lovers had more than affairs of the heart. They had sex that was "moore for delit than world to multiplye." And he wrote vociferously against any man who "putteth certeine material thynges in hire secree places" and "elles dooth unkyndely synne, by which men or womman shedeth hire nature seed in manere or in place ther as a child may nat be conceyved." Scholars always assumed this meant Chaucer was against the practice of abortion, but it might actually be Chaucer against the condom.

He and other writers of the Middle Ages and into the Renaissance unintentionally helped explain how, in spite of the fact that the nobility often flaunted extramarital and premarital affairs, pregnancy was notably absent in references to the benighted lovers who experimented with courtly love. But did the knights of the realm actually use armor other than the chain mail variety?

Although there is not a great deal of evidence that condom use was widespread or widely understood in the Middle Ages, there is plenty of evidence that many men worked hard to make sure that having sex, especially the illicit variety, would not have any nasty repercussions. The knights, as chivalrous, gallant, and worldly as they were, would have been aware of the methods they could use to spare their precious lamens the discomfort and embarrassing aftereffects of "delit." Hopefully none of them followed one very powerful birth control expert's advice.

A PAPAL RECOMMENDATION

A very interesting description of a male covering came from another clergyman, but this one was not tucked away in a scriptorium. He was a pope.

Pope John XXI was born Peter of Spain in the thirteenth century. The son of a physician, Pope John studied at the University of Paris and became a medical lecturer at the University of Siena. This doctor-pope wrote quite a bit about contraception. He cataloged the herbs women could use for birth control—*and* he called upon men to show restraint. But he also recommended a condom made out of a paste from the bark and leaves of the hemlock tree. Pope John, however, must have had a somewhat limited understanding of sex: his pasty condom covered the testicles, not the penis!

Another thirteenth-century sex expert, Antoninus, wrote about contraceptives in a pseudomedical treatise with the guilty title *Confessional of Antoninus*. The penitent writer spoke dramatically about his use of the "poisons of sterility," a common, Church-inspired phrase encompassing all contraceptives. But it is Antoninus's oblique reference to what men could do to prevent accidents that makes the somewhat whimsical (and very long) tract both telling and entertaining. The author referred to two ways men could have sex using a "vessel" made out of soft hide. Though it is very vague, he recommends having sex "outside the vessel" and "within the vessel." Like his fellows, Antoninus's language is veiled, but he leaves plenty of room to ponder the linguistic possibilities: condom versus "vessel." There is also the distinct possibility that Antoninus was neither anticontraception nor guilty.

PENIS CAPTIVUS

Although women had more freedom and choice during the Middle Ages, all was not rosy when it came to their treatment under Church and secular laws. Nowhere was this more evident than in the publication of the horrendous fourteenth-century tome Malleus Maleficarum (Witches' Hammer). The book warned men that witches lurked everywhere and that consorting with them could be deadly or at least uncomfortable, because a witch could "deprive man of his virile member." Other antiwoman treatises warned that intercourse could cause leprosy, and one foretold of what could be interpreted as a unique women's condom: "Some women are so wary and cunning that they take iron and place it in the vagina. This . . . wounds the penis . . ." It probably would not have done the vagina any good either.

Then there was the penis captivus, the medieval notion that once a man's member was "sucked in," he could not get away from the woman he was having sex with, snared in the missionary position for eternity. Another "trap" witchy, wily women could use was the aiguillette, a leather ligature that wrapped around the penis, condom-style. Originally meant as an aid to prevent men from hanging out while they rode long distances or played certain sports (and reminiscent of the Greek dog knot), it could be used by evildoers, too. Rather than trapping an unsuspecting sex partner into eternal sex, though, this thing was supposed to actually prevent a man from having sex at all—a sort of castrating condom. Definitely the work of witches.

WHAT WOULD LEONARDO HAVE DONE?
WAS THERE A RENAISSANCE FOR THE CONDOM?

As the Middle Ages progressed, the Catholic Church became more and more concerned about sex and how it related to sin. Yet the dichotomy remains that some of the most prolific birth control writers and experimenters were monks in the scriptoriums and friars in their parishes. And the many children running around the Vatican, sired by popes; the married priests with their behind-the-scenes families; and the generally lax attitude toward churchmen's sexual transgressions indicates that the married-only, sex-for-procreation message was not necessarily heeded even by insiders, let alone by the general populace. It also seems likely that the work of the busy monks in their scriptoriums was not read by some of their fellow churchmen, judging by the many illegitimate children of the clergy.

In spite of the fantastic advances realized in science and technology during the Renaissance, however, there were no major breakthroughs in birth control methods by the fifteenth century. It remained mostly the responsibility of women, who continued to take the same useful and useless potions of herbs their forebears had used, as well as employing a similar variety of pessaries and female condoms; the tampon dipped in strong liquids with spermicidal qualities was reborn after an absence of at least five hundred years.

The odd recommendations for salves and tar-based testicle and penis coverings also remained in the birth control repertoire of the citizen of the Renaissance. And, of course, there was always the magical amulet! But it was in the flourishing cities and towns of Europe, especially in England and France,

RENAISSANCE CHARMS

A popular contraceptive not taken internally, the heart of a salamander worn as a charm was believed to work wonders when it was pinned near a woman's knees. Another charm, known as a breve—a folded paper object containing powerful magic—may not have been as useful. When a brother gave an abbess he was sleeping with a breve, he instructed her to wear it on a silk thread around her neck while they were having sex, promising it would prevent "offspring." He had fled by the time she realized the breve had failed, which prompted the abbess to open up the charm. In bad Latin, it read, "Don't let yourself get laid, and you will not fill the cup."

where tradesmen who worked with animal by-products—and kept their knowledge close to their sleeves—knew how to make condoms ... and eventually how to market them.

> *"To which Diasakos did you go as a boy?"*
> *"I was educated by blows in the slaughterhouse."*
> *"What wrestling did you learn from the paid tribes?"*
> *"To steal and perjure myself and look the other way."*
> *'What technique did you have on coming to manhood?"*
> *"Sausage selling."*
>
> From the Athenian Aristophanes' play *The Knights*

SAUSAGE MAKERS AND GLOVERS

The word *sausage* is derived from the Latin *salcicia* meaning salted, probably because thanks to salt, sausage was one of humankind's first preserved foods; the salt and spices in early varieties, like those favored by Babylonian king Nebuchadnezzar, meant that sausages stayed fresh for a long time. The Romans even used their beloved *nenia* (small, spicy links) in religious ceremonies. A favorite Greek play from the fifth century BCE was simply titled *The Sausage*. Haggis (an old English, not Scottish Gaelic word) put the soupy kind of sausage on the map, and Homer even mentions sausages in his epic *The Odyssey*. And by the Middle Ages, the Italians had the biggest variety of sausage types ever; they still do. The sausage has quite a history and one that has had great influence on another little item.

The shape of both items is the first clue as to why the maker of one would figure out the use of the same material to make the other. Animal intestines—bladders, galls, skins—have been used to make condoms for thousands of years. The most popular high-quality sheath of the twenty-first century is still made from gut. Historians interested in the origins of modern commerce and specifically the reemergence of retail at the microlevel have for years been making the vague but enduring claim that slaughterhouse workers were the first in early modern Europe to invent or discover an alternative use for animal guts. Probably true, but it is also true that sausage makers themselves had a minor side trade in providing cleaned, treated material for individual sale and, by the sixteenth century, to people who made a living out of making condoms for retail sales.

Of course, the Europeans did not invent this alternative use, but it is likely that they thought they had. The fact that fewer than 3 percent of Europeans could read and write either in their own vernacular languages or in Latin is a good reason for the lack of clear and concise records in regard to who sold what, for how much, and to whom. And considering what a blush can be raised in the twenty-first century when the little device is mentioned, it is little wonder that sausage makers, butchers, or slaughter men did not pass on their knowledge about condoms in a public manner. They may also have feared the churchman and the taxman.

The sausage makers of Europe and England were busy men and women with their own guilds (the Venetian sausage guild rivaled the goldsmith guild for its rich endowments to the church of San Salvatore). They were also less regulated than standard butchers when it came to medieval law codes. In thirteenth- and fourteenth-century London, butchers were frequently fined for befouling streets and even the Thames River with their "offal, blood, and entrails." The sausage makers had no such worries. They bought their meats prepared, along with spices, salt, and animal bladders.

In London, bladders were available from specialty butchers who did a vigorous trade on Blow Bladder Street, immortalized by Daniel Defoe, the son of a butcher, in his *Journal of the Plague Year*. Since at least 1284, the sausage makers of Blow Bladder, or just Bladder, Street came to buy cleaned and prepared intestines in order to produce their own variety of meat product and for resale. And though the sausage makers did not leave any "receipts" for their version of the condom, they would have resembled earlier, primitive sheaths, but cut with meat cleavers, tied in a knot at one end to prevent leakage, and attached at the top with a ribbon or a string once on the wearer.

> *Well, hurry up! In you go, sausage,*
> *Nice and tight, the path is narrow . . .*
> *Don't pray tell: don't you love*
> *This illustrious and rich blood sausage*
> *How the treacherous one stings!*

It must be loaded with spices.
Spanish author Baltasar del Alcazar, seventeenth century

"HAND IN GLOVE . . ."

Long before Shakespeare (whose father was a glover) had Cressida hand her glove to Troilus, symbolizing the sex act, the glove had been used in literature as a double entendre, a symbol for both the penis and the vagina, one which spoke to both the role of women and the role of men in sex.

Glove making itself was a woman-friendly business during the Middle Ages, and women glovers had their own guilds. They also had a direct connection to slaughterhouse workers and butchers, because they used some of the same materials to produce gloves as those other professions. And they, too, held the wisdom of the bladder condom and how to produce it for personal use, as well as to make a bit on the side. Lesser glovers, those allowed by guild law to make only linen or wool gloves, were not considered to be true professionals and did not belong to the glovers' guilds. But they also used the same materials as the condom makers who preferred to produce linen sheaths—both used fabric and both were likely to finish off their products with strips of fabric or even ribbons.

Female glovers as well as the Jewish male glovers increasingly turned to condom manufacturing as the Middle Ages and the Renaissance gave way to the sixteenth century, a time when the European economy was changing rapidly and was not so tolerant of women in the world of trade. Gone were the days when women worked side by side with men, and gone were the women's guilds that had dignified and protected the glovers' profession. Women were pushed out of the business world, and those who remained often had to find outlets in fringe economies for their skills. Gloves to condoms was a logical move for some, and the women sausage makers suffered the same fate. By the seventeenth century, when condom makers were far more public than in the earlier years, most manufacturers who made condoms on a grand scale were women—and in Spain and Italy, a few Jewish men, who had been pushed into narrow "professional" roles during the anti-Semitic Middle Ages, fashioned *skins* to order.

Is it any wonder, then, that the three most enduring euphemisms for the condom are *bladder*, *skin*, and *glove*?

THREE

le male de naples, la mal françois, las bubas, or the venetian disease

COLUMBUS AND THE GREAT POX

By the early sixteenth century, select Europeans had gazed upon Botticelli's *Birth of Venus* and da Vinci's *Mona Lisa*. Lords and ladies enjoyed their first popular secular music, with madrigal singers and lute players much in demand, perhaps while they were also reading Pico della Mirandola's *Oration on the Dignity of Man* and Thomas Malory's *Morte d'Arthur*, the fictional work that introduced the enduring legend of King Arthur and his knights.

As early as 1430, a variety of type sets had been introduced by printers in Holland and Germany, making it possible for more than thirty-five thousand books to have been published by the year 1500, a far cry from the earlier labors of the monks in their scriptoriums. The English middle class was enjoying an increasing literacy rate, creating a large market for the mass-produced books, many of which were being printed on modern paper made from wood pulp, a brand-new process.

Even the toothbrush had been invented by 1498. Ah, yes, the Renaissance was truly a magical time.

But there was also a dark side to this brilliant era. Deadly political intrigue of the sort portrayed in Machiavelli's treatise *The Prince* was rife, leading to frequent and bloody squabbles between kings and princes over turf and trade, fights that in turn led to a series of petty wars between city-states and nations alike.

Despite the influences of brilliant men like Galileo and Copernicus, and the slow move toward enlightened thought that eventually led to the creation of humanism, citizens of Europe were still being burned at the stake for their scientific, political, and religious beliefs—or because they had been accused of cavorting with the devil.

It is in this tumultuous atmosphere that Europeans like Christopher Columbus launched their campaigns to explore the uncharted lands beyond their own continent. But their adventures and the rewards that accompanied the opening up of the globe came at a very high price for many. And this proved that necessity really is the mother of invention, or in this case, the condom.

A DISEASE PREVIOUSLY UNKNOWN

Biblical scholars believe that many of the leprous plagues mentioned in the Bible were actually references to venereal infections. After fighting with the Midianites, Israelite soldiers were ordered to execute all Midianite women prisoners "that have known man by lying with him." Leviticus 14 advises washing after copulation. Beyond that, though Romans used the condom for protection against prostitutes' *spurcae* and *Mount Vesuvius's rash*, the ancients and early Europeans rarely referred specifically to sexually trans-mitted infections—until 1495.

TRACTADO CONTRA EL MAL SERPENTINA

From Treatise against the Evil Snake: *"The reason I call it serpentine is because one cannot find a more horrible comparison, for as this animal is hideous, dangerous and terrible." Snakes were associated with the phallus; Diaz de Isla equated the poison of a syphilitic's penis with the venom of a snake.*

*A mysterious epidemic, hitherto unknown, which had struck terror
into all hearts by the rapidity of its spread, the ravages it made, and
the apparent helplessness of the physicians to cure it.*

A sixteenth-century chronicler

Upon their return from Haiti, Columbus's Spanish sailors sought medical treatment in Barcelona from physician Ruy Diaz de Isla, who later published the very first account of what he dubbed the *Indian measles*, a "disease, previously unknown, unseen and undescribed which spread thence throughout the world."

After treatment, the sailors left Barcelona to sell their services as mercenaries to the Spanish and French forces fighting over control of the kingdom of Naples. French king Charles VIII's army was attempting to claim Naples for the French crown, a plan that included Charles's grander intention of becoming Emperor of the East. In response, King Ferdinand V of Castile sent his own army to help his kinsman King Ferdinand II of Naples to repel the intended French invasion.

When they arrived in Italy, the contagious sailor-mercenaries went straight to the Neapolitan brothels, where they infected the prostitutes, who then moved on to service other soldiers—Castilian, French, and Italian. The Indian measles, which seems to have become more virulent as it traveled, spread like wildfire throughout the ranks of both camps, and then into the city, transmitting the mysterious disease to more than half of the civilian population.

Europe's first epidemic of what is now called the great pox slammed Naples in 1495, only a few years after Columbus's return from the New World. In its wake, instead of Charles becoming Emperor of the East, his foolish quest was dashed before it had really begun: his army, a ragtag collection of mercenaries from all over Europe, had been destroyed by superior forces, Charles's royal ineptitude, and disease.

That was not the end for either the disease or the Spanish mercenaries, however. Some of those who survived headed to Scotland that same year, where they offered their services to King James IV and to an English pretender trying to claim the throne of Scotland. While James and the pretender battled it out over who would rule, Edinburgh was hit hard by an epidemic of the great pox, brought by the same mercenaries. James, trying to "combat the infirmity come out of France and strange parts," commanded "that all light women to desist from their vices and sin of venerie" (demonstrating the fact that he understood that the contagion was somehow related to sex). He also passed a law that included punishing with a distinctive brand on the cheek anyone thought to be infected with the pox. In spite of the heavy penalties, the disease continued to spread, and was so feared that James decreed that any Scot who had it would be banished to the remote Scottish island of Inch. The boat left every Friday, full of sufferers.

As evidenced by the Edinburgh epidemic, when the Spanish mercenaries exited Naples, they took the new disease with them, spreading it throughout Europe and beyond. As the pox moved from place to place, it was identified with the country from which it was assumed to have originated. The Italians called it the *Spanish disease*, the English called it the *French pox*, the Spanish called it the *Castilian disease*, the Poles named it after the Russians, and the Russians named it after the Poles. By 1505, the *Christian, Polish, French, Neapolitan, Russian, Spanish, Persian, Turkish, English pox* had traveled all the way to Asia. Other appellations included *las bubas, bosen blattern, mankabassam, malade Frantzos,* and *Cupid's measles.* But by the sixteenth century, the terrible disease was known to most simply as *syphilis.*

> **VOLTAIRE**
> The first fruit the Spaniards brought from the New World was syphilis.

> **SURELY THE WORK OF WITCHES**
> An English euphemism for the pox also included the Occult Disease, blaming witches for the contagion.

SYPHILIS SIVE MORBUS GALLICUS: "SYPHILIS, OR THE FRENCH DISEASE"

Sixteenth-century Italian humanist, physician, scientist, and poet Girolamo Fracastoro actually gave *syphilis* its name. Friend and colleague of Coper-

De Morbo Gallico. 52

uerucam, & mediam partem glandis exesit: sed quia ego dixi quòd caries oritur per contagium. sciatis quòd etiam oriri solet ratione hepatis transmittentis: dimittamus hanc secundam speciem loquamur de prima, atque quo iuuenis coiens cum infecta ab hac præseruetur, & cariem non sentiat.

De præseruatione à carie Gallica.   CAP. LXXXVIIII.

Ego nihil fecisse uideor nisi doceam uos, quomodo quis uidens pulcherrimam sirenam, & coiens cum ea, etiam infecta, à carie, & lue Gallica præseruetur. Ego semper fui huius sententiæ, quòd adsit ratio præcauendi, ne per contagium, huiusmodi ulcera oriantur: sed quæ est ista ratio? Ego dixi quòd nascitur caries hæc per communicata corpuscula saniosa, quæ imbibita poris glandis faciunt cariem, ideò opus est, ut statim saniem à glande expurgemus, sed si imbibita sit in poris licet uino, lotio, uel aqua detergamus priapum, tamen eam detergere non possumus. & hoc sæpe accidit in tectis, & mollibus glandibus. Quomodo ergo agendum? semper fui istius sententiæ, quòd ponamus aliquod habens uim penetrandi corium, & dissipandæ materiæ, uel extrahendæ, uel siccandæ & uincendæ natura sua. ideò inuestigaui hoc medicamentum. Sed quia oportet etiam Meretricum animos disponere, non licet nobiscum unguenta domo afferre. propterea ego inueni linteolum imbutum medicamento, quod potest commodè asportari, cum fæmoralia iam ita uasta feratis, ut totam apotecam uobiscum habere possitis: Quoties ergo quis coiuerit abluat (si potest) pudendum, uel panno detergat: postea habeat linteolum ad mensuram glandis præparatum; demum cum coiuerit ponat supra glandem, & recurrat præputium: si potest madere sputo, uel lotio bonum est, tamen non refert: si timetis, ne caries oriatur in medio canali, habeatis huius lintei inuolucrium, & in canali ponatis, ego feci experimentum in centum, & mille hominibus, & Deum testor immortalem nullum eorum infectum. Notate autem obiter, quòd quælibet species lienteoli mundi tantam habet uim in præseruatione, ut nihil magis [addite quòd gossipium nouum, molle, fidibus bene concussum glandi optimè lotæ detergentibus, obuolutum mirum in modù præseruat, & quum quis Gallicis scopulis lignum percussit post ablationem inspiciat: uidebit enim inuolucrium illud saniosum, aut citrino, aut pallido, uel subnigro colore infectum] ideò semper quis paruo linteolo obuoluat glandem per spatium quatuor, aut quinque horarum, & hoc non est molestum mulieribus: sed tamen præparati lintei ratio est præstantissima. Præparatur autem hoc modo.

Nota de præseruatione.

Lotio ex vino et Vino.

Linteolum mundum. Gossipiu.

Præparatio lintei.

De Morbo Gallico: "The French Disease"

RENAISSANCE FRACASTORO'S POETRY

To Naples first it came
from France, and justly took
from France his hame
Companion from the war . . .

To whom all Indian Traffick is unknown
Nor could th' infection from the
Western Clime
Seize distant nations at the
self same time.

If then by Traffick thence this
plague was brought
How dearly was that
Traffick bout!

Nor can th' infection first be
charged on Spain
That sought new worlds beyond
the Western main.
Since from Pyrene's foot, to Italy
It shed its bane on France,
while Spain was free.
From whence 'tis plain this Pest
must be assign'd
To some more pow'rful cause and
hard to find.

Since nature's then so liable to change
Why should we think this late
contagion strange?

The offices of nature to define
And to each cause a true effect assign
Must be a task both hard
and doubtful too.

. . . nature always to herself
is true.

At first approach of Spring,
I would advise,
or ev'n in Autumn months
if strength suffice,
To bleed your patient in the regal vein,
And by degrees th' infected
current drain.

Nor let the foulness of the
course displease.
Obscene indeed, but less than
your disease.

The mass of humors now dissolved within,
To purge themselves by spittle shall begin,
Till you with wonder at your feet shall see,
A tide of filth, and bless the remedy.

A sheperd once (distrust not
ancient fame)
Possessed these downs, and
Syphilus his name
A thousand heifers in these vales he fed,
A thousand ewes to those fair rivers led.

This drought our Syphilus beheld with pain,
Nor could the sufferings of his
flock sustain,
But to the noonday sun with
upcast eyes,
In rage threw these reproaching
blasphemies. . . .

nicus and professor of logic at the University of Padua, Fracastoro was the first academic to posit the cause of epidemics in relation to disease and was convinced that syphilis—like other deadly contagions—was transferable through seedlike entities, transmitting infection directly or indirectly, from host to host. Fascinated by the deadly contagion, Fracastoro also wrote an epic poem about the *French disease*, renaming the contagion after his own mythic shepherd, *Syphylus*.

Borrowing from Greek legend, Fracastoro told of a young shepherd from Atlantis who was punished by Apollo for worshiping other gods. The punishment was that Syphylus (both spellings appear in Fracastoro's work and in later translations) suffered from ulcers all over his body.

The origins of the shepherd's name are debatable. It is possible Fracastoro borrowed it from Sipylus, a character in Ovid's *Metamorphoses*, but whatever its provenance, the term *syphilis* undoubtedly caught on in part because it did not point the finger at any one group, country, or culture. Despite that, the poem does provide a fascinating look, not

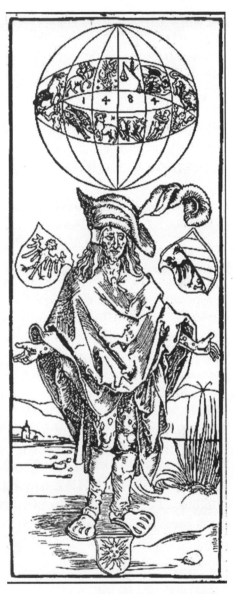

Albrecht Dürer's Syphilitic

just at the early history of the spread of a deadly, sexually transmitted disease, but at the politics of the times.

Fracastoro rightfully accused the Spanish of introducing the disease, only to avoid the consequences of its spread: "Since from Pyrene's foot to Italy . . . [i]t shed its bane on France . . . while Spain was free."

PINK RIBBONS AND A LINEN SHEATH— THE FIRST MODERN CONDOM

Grind the wood. Boil in water. Drink. Lock yourself in a heated,
sealed room or chamber, and sweat out the ill-humours.
An early sixteenth-century cure for the French disease

Throughout the sixteenth century, syphilis continued to spread across Europe and around the world: quacks were everywhere, happily preying on desperate victims, selling cures in the form of recipes, poultices, amulets, and prayers. Some of the cures were benign, others almost as deadly as the disease itself. But it took more than sixty years after the first epidemic for a European to contemplate a preventative to syphilis.

Gabriello Fallopio, another Italian academic, is the anatomist credited with discovering the Fallopian tube. He also wrote a treatise on syphilis, *De Morbo Gallico*, published posthumously in 1564, two years after his death. In it he described the first modern condom, which he claimed to have invented.

Although sheaths had been around for thousands of years prior to the printing of *De Morbo Gallico*, the written evidence that early modern Europeans used "conventional" male barriers was buried in ancient text, innu-

FALLOPIO'S PHALLUS FANTASIES

Fallopio recommended to parents of baby boys that they "take every pain in infancy to enlarge the privy member of boys, since a well-grown specimen never comes amiss." He did not go into detail as to how parents were to accomplish this.

endo, and trade secrets, so it is likely Fallopio really did believe he had invented the condom.

What Fallopio describes in his book is a piece of linen, sewn together to fit just the glans of the penis. The early version did not sound terribly comfortable, but according to Fallopio it did what he had designed it to do—it prevented men from becoming infected with a venereal disease, specifically syphilis.

According to Fallopio, "As often as a man has intercourse, he should (if possible) wash the genitals, or wipe them with a cloth; afterward he should use a small linen cloth made to the glans, and draw forward the prepuce over the glans; if he can do so, it is well to moisten it with saliva or with a lotion. . . . I tried the experiment on eleven hundred men, and I call immortal God to witness that not one of them was infected." He also recommended an alternative way to wear his condom: inserted into the urethra. It is doubtful many men availed themselves of this uncomfortable alternative application, however.

Fallopio obviously made the connection between covering the man's member and disease prevention: he believed that the "fluids" swapped between the man and the woman were directly connected to contagion. With that in mind, he also soaked his condoms in a chemical solution, which inadvertently acted as a spermicide—a technique that would remain popular for hundreds of years. Fallopio's goal was to keep men safe from disease; he kept no records on the women with whom his subjects had had sex. If he had, his second realization might have been that the *Fallopian condom* was also a birth control device.

Fallopio did at least think of women when he made one concession to feminine tastes: he had pink silk ribbons sewn on to hold them in place, with the ribbon tied around the shaft of the penis. He was quite proud of that flourish—one he very likely learned from the women who made the sheaths for him, though claiming the whole thing as his brainchild—as well as the convenience of his invention, which could be hidden away in a purse or a pocket until needed.

When news of Fallopio's humble little condom spread, gone were the days of "hinting" at its existence and purpose, as it appeared in a variety of literary genres: medical, political, and religious. By the end of the sixteenth century, Hercules of Saxonia wrote about a disease-preventing "sheath" made of linen, dipped in a chemical solution and allowed to dry. But it was at the same time that French writer Leonard Lessius, in his book *Law and Justice*,

> ## A SIXTEENTH-CENTURY JESUIT'S CONDEMNATION
> *. . . or anything else to prevent conception, is guilty of mortal sin against nature. This sin cannot be erased by any good intention. This is in fact deliberately impeding the seed from realizing its natural purpose, which is procreation, and this differs little from ejaculation outside the natural receptacle: it is only a question of degree . . .*
>
> Brother Tomas Sanchez might have known about condoms. He certainly understood that Christians were practicing birth control.

referred to the use of the condom as immoral, which indicates that though Fallopio had been slow to realize it, the modern condom had immediately crossed over from the only thing coming between lovers and disease . . . to once again being recognized (or acknowledged) as birth control.

Either way, the fantastic new invention traveled swiftly throughout Europe, across the English Channel, and around the world.

CLOTHING AND THE CONDOM—
THE CODPIECE—PRETTY OR PRACTICAL?

A precursor to and first cousin of Fallopio's linen condom, and one that was considerably more public, is the codpiece.

Similar to the genesis of the ancient Egyptian and Greek sheath from clothing to protection, the codpiece grew out of some major fashion changes under way by the mid-fourteenth century. Initially, young men who spent a lot of time on horseback and those who served in the armies began to shorten their tunics for convenience and comfort. No flowing robes or long jackets to get tangled up in.

This shortening trend became so extreme that some men's costumes

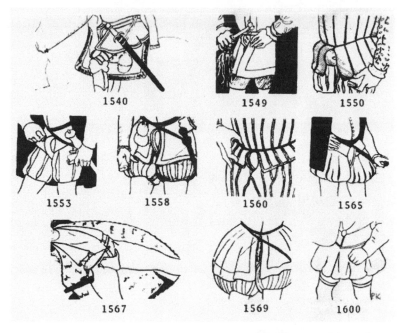

Evolution of the codpiece

dwindled to hose and very short chemises. These trendy gentlemen were so likely to "hang out" of their scant clothing that England's rather prudish King Edward IV became very concerned on moral—and visual—grounds. He ordered that when a man came to his court, he had to wear some kind of jacket to "cover his privy members and buttockkes." This led to a series of tricky styles for flaplike coverings made to hide the offending penises, which quickly evolved into separate items of clothing, and definitely *objectified* the male member.

It was after the late fifteenth-century syphilis outbreaks, however, that the real codpiece appeared. Taking its lead from the fashion trend dictating less is more, the true codpiece was a hollow, layered box made in various shapes and sizes, often with sumptuous fabrics decorating the outside. The

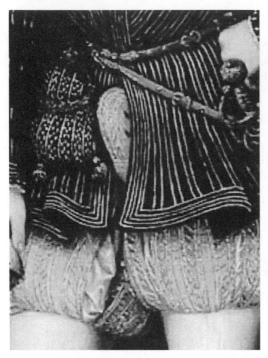

*Dressing for success:
A seventeenth-century
gentleman*

interior fabric lining these sheaths was usually soft linen, probably removable for washing. Different styles sported a variety of methods in which to attach the codpiece to the wearer, much like ancient penis sheaths; and of course they had to be easy to remove in order to answer nature's call.

But what was the codpiece's relationship to syphilis? Clothing historians have pondered the true meaning of the codpiece, claiming everything from symbolic phallic worship at a time of extreme machismo in fashion history to an interesting variation of a purse. In fact, evidence points to the codpiece's evolution as a boxy sheath for protection—protection from prying eyes, painful blows, and stained clothing.

The ointments used to relieve the pain of syphilitic infection turned the penis bright orange. To be seen with the telltale orange unguent was a social disgrace, because it proved the man had syphilis, a guaranteed way to find himself socially ostracized (in spite of the many noblemen with the disease). It also protected the outer clothing from being stained by oozing sores and messy medications. More important, this disease made a man's member very, very tender and painful. The codpiece, with its many layers and boxy, roomy nature, provided excellent protection from being jostled in a crowd and bumped by the accoutrements the average man of the late

Renaissance carried on his belt—purses, swords, daggers, and so forth. Only when men's clothing styles changed and once again became more modest did the codpiece—or the need for it—disappear.

CHAUCER'S TAKE ON CODPIECES

Alas! some of them show the very boss of the penis and the horrible pushed-out testicles that look like the malady of hernia in the wrapping of their hose, and the buttocks of such persons look like the hinder parts of a she-ape in the full of the moon. And moreover, the hateful proud members that they show by the fantastic fashion of making one leg of their hose white and the other red, make it seem that half of their privy members are flayed. And if it be that they divide their hose in other colours, as white and black, or white and blue, or black and red, and so forth, then it seems, by the variation of colour, that the half of their privy members are corrupted by the fire of Saint Anthony, or by cancer, or by other such misfortune.

On the codpiece, a not very sexy description by Chaucer's Parson

POSTURES AND THE ANCIENT ART OF PAPER FOLDING: WHAT ABOUT THE EXOTIC EAST?

European explorers had been working to establish trade relations in Asia since Marco Polo's time. By the fifteenth century, intrepid sailors and traders continued to forge strong import-export ties in China, India, and Japan, trading European-made wares for beautiful silks and other exotic goods highly valued at home. But the Westerners also brought something else to the Orient: they arrived carrying a new disease.

Syphilis had reached China and Japan by the beginning of the sixteenth century, and India in the late fifteenth century. By the 1700s, even the remote islands of the South Pacific were affected.

But did the peoples of the East use condoms—whether for protection from disease or for birth control—by or prior to the fifteenth century? The simple answer is yes.

Chinese condoms, *yin-chia*, were alternately made from oiled silk, paper, and lamb intestines. Like its early European linen counterparts, the yin-chia covered only the very top of the man's penis and was used mostly by the idle rich, men who enjoyed the kind of exotic sexual encounters described in erotic Chinese writings but who did not want to suffer the consequences of unexpected pregnancies. Sexually transmitted infections do not really seem to have been a consideration, mainly because the Chinese were generally very careful about personal hygiene. In fact, there was one universally accepted way in which to maintain cleanliness, common throughout the country: Chinese men and women were careful to wash their private parts both before and after sex. If there were any small wounds or abrasions, they rubbed a jelly made from agar-agar on their genitals to prevent any spread of infection.

THE PLUMS OF CANTON

It is believed that the Chinese did suffer from nonlethal variations of sexually transmitted infections prior to the sixteenth century, but they were never a huge health risk—until the world-traveling Europeans introduced the dreaded pox.

Known to them as *Cantonese sores* or *plum-blossom sores*, syphilis had decimated large areas of the country—central China was hardest hit—by the second quarter of the 1600s. And it did not take long for the medical experts of the time to associate sex with the spread of the awful disease. That knowledge and understanding did not extend to the common people, however, who (not unlike the average European) blamed the disease on all sorts of real and imagined sources. They figured it was just another possible way in which to die a miserable death, lumping it together with smallpox, the plague, and other threats to the daily existence of a Chinese peasant. But the use of the yin-chia among the upper classes helped them avert infection when syphilis hit.

PORTUGUESE POX

By the late fifteenth century, the Japanese also suffered from an outbreak of syphilis, which they called *mankabassam* (the *Portuguese sickness*), so named because they believed—accurately so—that it was Vasco de Gama's Portuguese sailors who had brought the disease to Japan. The spread of this terrible contagion coincided with the introduction of a European-style condom, the *kawa-gata* or *mara-bukuro*: penis sack. It was made from fine leather and introduced to the Japanese by Dutch traders.

Prior to the appearance of syphilis, the Japanese had used the *Kabuto-gata* (helmet) for birth control. The helmet was made from very thin, decoratively carved tortoise shell or animal horns. But the sack was much more comfortable for men than the Kabuto-gata, though women were said to have preferred the traditional helmet for its firmness. Either way, syphilis meant the condom served two purposes in Japanese society, as birth control and as disease prevention.

SEAGULLS AND STEEDS

Both in Japan and in China, there were books devoted to the sexual act, and its many possible variations. The Japanese versions included very imaginative descriptions of sexual postures or positions. Couples had plenty of options to choose from: the *flying seagulls*, the *galloping steed*, the *winding dragon*, the *fluttering butterflies*, *bamboos near the altar*, the *two dancing female phoenix birds*, to name a few. There is evidence that as condom use became more prevalent among the Japanese, its use was incorporated into the rituals involved in the choice of sexual postures. Putting on the penis sack was treated as a sort of foreplay, slipping on the kawa-gata as the couple got into position. The postures, however, may have been inspired by a much earlier source.

In eighth-century Japan, Shinto priests used the venerable art of paper folding to make a truly amazing condom. A relative of origami, the art of *kokigami* was the celibate priests' contribution to art and to the history of the condom. Elaborately folded into shapes of exotic, ferocious, and virile animals such as tigers, bears, and lions, the paper condoms were meant to bring out the beast in any man.

The wearer was instructed to picture himself as the animal he was wearing while he and his partner acted out the appropriate fantasies during sex (for the unimaginative, the paper condoms came with prefab scripts written by the priests). There is no way to tell quite what happened to the kokigami when the games began, but there was nothing humble about this condom!

THE KAMA SUTRA

Although syphilis had reached India by the end of the 1490s, Indians' use of the condom does not seem to intersect with disease prevention or birth control, but it does predate the arrival of syphilis. In his eighth-century (CE) sexual advice book *The Kama Sutra*, Dama Sutra of Vatsysyana talks about positions, stimulants, and *apadravyas*—condoms.

Some historians believe the apadravya was similar to the Egyptian strap-on condom, meant to enhance the look (and size) of the penis, and to provide plenty of stimulation for the woman. And the uncomfortable (for the man) materials Dama Sutra recommended—wood, copper, silver, ivory, and gold—corroborate this view. But he also describes leather and buffalo horn condoms, both popular in Japan, which leaves the purpose of the Indian condom open to speculation, as do the descriptions of the three types of apadravyas Dama Sutra describes.

The first is the *armlet*, which "should be the same size as the lingam [penis], and should have its outer surface made rough with glob-

> ## SYPHILITIC LEPROSY
> By the eighteenth century, "lock" hospitals had been established in England and France. These facilities started in the Middle Ages as leprosarias, but the problem of what to do with dying syphilitics became so acute, the hospitals, which were little more than prisons, became a dumping ground for victims of the disease. They also illustrate the age-old association between leprosy and sexually transmitted infection: lock is a corruption of the French word loques, meaning rags, as it was the poor who suffered the cruel fate of ending up in these hospitals.

ules." Then there was the *couple*, which was made up of "two *armlets* put together." And finally, the *bracelet*, which was "three armlets joined together until they come up to the required length of the lingam."

The traditional interpretation of these devices is that they were intended to be worn by men struggling to satisfy hard-to-please women. But it is possible that the armlet, the couple, and the bracelet were meant to serve a more practical purpose. Either way, the Eastern cultures were in many ways far ahead of the West when it came to inventiveness and creativity—and the humble condom.

FOUR

may prick nor purse never fail you . . .

PARLIAMENTARIANS, POETS,
PUNDITS, AND PROVENANCE

Many historians have dubbed the seventeenth century the "century of war," an era when European leaders were using innovative new technologies to produce ever-more powerful weaponry in their competition for land, wealth, and power. The Thirty Years' War was one of many fought at this time, and just the name gives some clue as to the length of time men spent brutalizing their neighbors. The eighteenth century differed little, as the French Revolution proved just how cruel people could be toward their own. But like most other ages and eras in Western history, these were also times of great hope and intellectual development.

As Sir Isaac Newton discovered calculus, John Milton defended the freedom of the press, and John Locke suggested that the way to peace and prosperity for all was religious tolerance. The brave scientists and philosophers who still faced the possibility of cruel punishment for suggesting radical or irreligious ideas continued to promote the notion that reason rather than war and violence could win against ignorance, want, superstition, and tyrannical leadership.

Less exalted but important events and quirky trends also mark this as an exhilarating time in history: newspapers became available in major cities all over Europe, replacing the old weekly broadsheets; Stradivarius began making his violins; Parisians were using the self-loaded ink pen by 1657; and women's skirts were getting bigger and more elaborate, while men wore lots of leather and lace. And the arts and literature blossomed.

Cervantes's *Don Quixote de la Mancha* made its debut in Spain in 1615 and Parisians danced to the new Minuet; English poetry lovers elected John Dryden as their first poet laureate, and Shakespeare's *Othello, Measure for Measure*, and *All's Well That Ends Well* were performed at his Globe theater in London. In 1631 women finally broke the age-old "no woman rule" and appeared on the English stage, while Italian Francesca Caccini became the first woman to direct an opera.

Eventually, this brilliant, eccentric, and eclectic era was simply dubbed the Enlightenment. The condom thrived.

In spite of the lingering threat of disease and infection, life during the seventeenth and eighteenth centuries was anything but chaste, especially for the well-to-do. Along with the high-minded treatises by the great minds of the Enlightenment, there were also books, plays, poetry, and private diaries full of anecdotes about interesting sexual encounters. These provide snapshots of the more lascivious side of European life, and prove that the condom had by this time become so vital a component in the intimate lives of many, it was featured in some surprisingly public literary venues.

ROBINET AND SUSANNE

L'Escole des Filles (The Philosophy of Girls) was a bawdy book that did double duty as pornography and sex manual. Written by an anonymous Frenchman and first printed in Paris in 1655, the author described in lurid detail an unusual prop. The hero of the tale wore his condom proudly.

As he put it on, lover Robinet listened to his intimate friend Susanne talk about how amazing it was that a simple little piece of fabric made of linen and tied around his member with a silk ribbon could "catch the seed." Although the book was publicly condemned as obscene and reportedly

WORLD'S OLDEST CONDOM

Possibly the oldest surviving condom was made to be reusable and dates back to 1640. This pig intestine device comes from Sweden and was found with its original user's manual, written in Latin. The manual suggests the item be soaked in warm milk before using, which was supposed to help prevent disease.

popular only with the lower classes—who could not have afforded it or been able to read it—copies of it were in great demand among the nobility, especially the ladies of the court.

In the same year it was published as a novel, *L'Escole des Filles* was produced as a play, opening to packed audiences in Paris and other major French city centers. In the live version (surely X-rated), the condom was not left out of the plot. In fact, in one scene it played a conspicuous role, with Robinet donning *un petit linge* (a small cloth) in front of titillated audiences. While Robinet slowly put on his condom, Susanne turned to the audience and extolled the virtues of *un petit linge*—as a birth control device. Not only was this rowdy content for a seventeenth-century (or a twenty-first-century) play, it is probably the earliest Western literary reference to the condom as a contraceptive.

QUANDOM, CONDUM, CONDOM, CONDON, CONTON— DOCTOR OR COLONEL?

> *A Gut the Learn'd call, Blind;*
> *'Till Condon, for the great invention fam'd,*
> *Found out its Use, and after him 'twas nam'd.*

In spite of the fact that shortly after Fallopio's experiment, public knowledge of the condom had spread quickly across Europe, just the word *condom* illustrates that poor Fallopio was never really credited with his brilliant invention. Men do not put on a *fallopio* prior to having sex, and the Italian anatomist's contribution to public health has been all but lost to history. It is usually the English who were credited—or blamed—with inventing the little sheath.

In 1666, the year of the Great Fire of London, the English Birth Rate Commission officially documented the condom's popular use throughout the country by explaining that the significant decrease in births at the time was due to the use of "condons." This is the first time that spelling, or anything close to it, was used in an official government document.

Although the true etymology of the word is not and will likely never be known, the most persistent tradition explaining the origins of the word *condom* in all its varietal spellings grew up around England's King Charles II. The King Charles's condom legends have survived to the present day.

The story goes that the little device was actually the invention of a seventeenth-century royal physician, Dr. Condum, who served Charles II as his personal surgeon. In some versions of the legend, he was also referred to as Colonel Condum. King Charles was deeply concerned about his army contracting the "clap" (a term coined in the seventeenth century, describing all sexually transmitted infections, but later associated specifically with gonorrhea), fearing a major contagion could spoil his chances of regaining the English throne. Knowing he could never force abstinence upon his fighting men, Charles asked his personal surgeon to find a way to prevent infection. After the good doctor, or colonel, designed a linen sheath, complete with silk ribbon, the king had all his soldiers supplied with the new invention.

The legend goes on to say that Charles also had the colonel provide the royal's promiscuous aristocrats with the little items, hoping to limit the number of illegitimate children running around his court. One version of the story also says that poor Dr. Condum was so embarrassed by his newfound fame—and notoriety—that he had to change his distinctive name and go underground, never to be heard from again.

Strangely, the oldest preserved con-

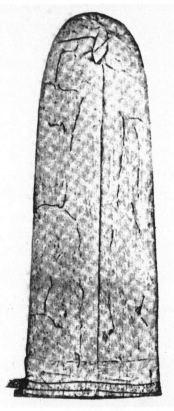

A seventeenth-century fish bladder sheath

THE *TATLER*

The legend of Dr. Condum or Colonel Condum persisted for centuries and was even featured in one of London's favorite eighteenth-century gossip sheets. In 1709 the Tatler printed a story about the good doctor enjoying a rare public appearance in a favorite watering hole, Will's Coffee House:

There are considerable Men [who] appear in all Ages, who for some eminent Quality or Invention, deserve the Esteem and Thanks of the Publick. Such a Benefactor is a Gentle-man of the House, who is observed by the Surgeons with Application, made it an Immodesty to name his Name. This Act of Self-denial has gain'd this worthy Member of the Commonwealth a great Reputation. Some law-givers have departed from the Abodes for ever, and commanded the Observation of their Laws till their Return; others have us'd other Artifices to fly the Applause of their Merit; but this Person shuns Glory with greater Address, and has by giving his Engine his own Name, made it ob-scene to speak of him more. However, he is rank'd among, and received by the modern Wits, as a Promoter of Gal-lantry and Pleasure.

doms from the seventeenth century did belong to the officers of Charles's father, Charles I. These sexual artifacts were found in a privy in the English Midlands' Castle Dudley. During the English Revolution of the 1640s, it appears the royalist officers had their last fling the night before a big battle fought on and around the grounds of the castle. Since they chose to protect themselves with their fish and animal bladder (not linen) condoms, they must have expected to win. Their caution was unnecessary, however, as Charles's army was routed that day, and the officers did not survive to appreciate the benefits of their precautions, though their paramours must have been grateful.

Although it is true the condom traveled around Europe, across the English Channel, and back again—and Charles did want to keep his army and his royals safe from disease and unwanted "bastards"—there was no Dr. Condum. First, the modern origins of the condom

WEBSTER'S ETYMOLOGY
Some legends are more persistent than others. The New Lexicon Webster's Dictionary of the English Language still refers to the story of Dr. Condum in its etymology for the modern word.

COFFEE AND CONDOMS

Coffeehouses were a new and exotic idea in the seventeenth century, and offered another quiet outlet for condom salespeople of the time. It is probable that these trendy shops were where Charles's officers picked up their supplies of fish gut engines.

A contemporary description of the new craze:

Adown the Strand, Fleet Street, and in that part of the city adjoining the Exchange, coffee-houses abounded in great numbers. Coffee, which in this reign became a favourite beverage, was introduced into London a couple of years before the restoration. It had, however, been brought into England at a much earlier period. John Evelyn, in the year 1638, speaks of it being drunk at Oxford, where there came to his college "one Nathaniel Conoposis out of Greece, from Cyrill the patriarch of Constantinople, who, returning many years after, was made Bishop of Smyrna." Twelve good years later, a coffee-house was opened at Oxford by one Jacobs, a Jew, where this beverage was imbibed "by some who delighted in novelty." It was, however, according to Oldys the antiquarian, untasted in the capital till a Turkey merchant named Edwards brought to London a Ragusan youth named Pasqua Rosee, who prepared this drink for him daily. The eagerness to taste the strange beverage drawing too much company to his board, Edwards allowed the lad, together with a servant of his son-in-law, to sell it publicly; whence coffee was first sold in St. Michael's Alley in Cornhill by Pasqua Rosee, "at the sign of his own head," about the year 1658.

Though coffee-drinkers first met with much ridicule from wits about town, and writers of broadsheet ballads, the beverage became gradually popular, and houses for its sale quickly multiplied. Famous amongst these, in the reign of the merry monarch, besides that already mentioned, was Garraway's in Exchange Alley; the Rainbow, by the Inner Temple Gate; Dick's, situated at No. 8, Fleet Street; Jacobs', the proprietor of which moved in 1671 from Oxford to Southampton Buildings, Holborn; the Grecian in the Strand, "conducted without ostentation or noise"; the Westminster, noted as a resort of peers and members of parliament; and Will's, in Russell Street, frequented by the poet Dryden.

lie in Italy. Second, condom is not, in any of its creative spellings, an English surname.

So where does the word come from? There are a number of medieval Latinate words that may provide clues: *condus* means both "preserve" and "receptacle," reflecting the fact that the original intent for the little device was to "preserve" the wearer from disease and that it was a receptacle for the "seed." Then there is *conduma*, meaning house (*con* or *cum* means "with"—*doma* or *duma* means "roof of a house") or even *cumdum*, which is either a false scabbard worn over a sword or the oilskin case for holding the colors of a military regiment.

Condus, *conduma*, or *cumdum* ... whatever the provenance, the legends are a fascinating addition to the history of euphemisms for the humble little condom.

SHAKESPEARE'S GLOVE AND THE POETIC QUONDAM

Especially in sixteenth- and seventeenth-century Scottish English, there were a lot of common idiomatic and slang words that were associated with sex and many began with *qu* (pronounced *k*), which replaced the *c* in more standard English spellings. Words like *quipped*, meaning a man's genitalia, *quaedam*, a common prostitute, and *quaint*, which Chaucer used extensively in "The Wife of Bath's Tale" to describe a woman's "privy" parts, is just a short list of

SHAKESPEARE'S GLOVE

Glove *has been a common euphemism for the condom for over five hundred years, and symbolic of sex since Shakespeare's day. Fictional literature from the Renaissance to the seventeenth century "fetishized" the glove, with male lovers depicted as secretly obtaining the object of their affection's glove, fanaticizing about who put what into where.*

An exiled Spanish courtier, living at Elizabeth I's court, wrote to a lady he admired:

I have been so troubled not to have at hand the dog's skin gloves your ladyship desires that, pending the time when they shall arrive, I have resolved to sacrifice myself to your service and flay a piece of my own skin from the most tender part of my body, if such an uncouth carcass as mine can have any tender skin. To this length can love and the wish to serve a lady be carried that a man should flay himself to make gloves for this lady out of his own skin. But in my case this is nothing, for even my soul will skin itself for the person it loves. If my soul were visible like my body, the most pitiful soul would be seen and the most pitiful thing that has ever been looked upon. The gloves, my lady, are made of dog's skin, though they are mine; for I hold myself a dog and beg your ladyship to keep me in your service upon the honour and love of a faithful dog.

sexy *qu* words. However, the most interesting, *quondam*, appears in Western literature's most important works, strongly suggesting the possibility of a Shakespearean condom.

> ## THE BARD'S FATHER
> *John Shakespeare, the Bard's father, is said to have sold some of the finest* skinnes—gloves—*in Stratford.*

It seems more than probable that Will Shakespeare, a man with a profound sense of his own times, would have known about condoms and their increasing usage during his lifetime. He would also have been exposed to them as a soldier while serving in Flanders. Either way, it seems very likely he may have cleverly incorporated the little item into some of his best comic and sexually charged dialogue.

For instance, in some editions of *Henry V*, the character Pizzle (old English slang for penis) is married to Mistress Quickly. Pizzle (sometimes spelled Pistol) says of his new wife, "I have and I will hold the quondam Quickly," perhaps inferring the childless couple intended to remain that way.

In *Troilus and Cressida*, Shakespeare again used quondam, and he introduced the word glove, which was a common condom euphemism at the time, and one that is still in use today. Hector's cleverly paired words certainly suggest more than something worn on the hand:

> *O, you my lord! by Mars his gauntlet, thanks!*
> *Mock not, that I affect the untraded oath;*
> *Your quondam wife swears still by Venus' glove . . .*

Mars and Venus were unmarried lovers. The gauntlet . . . glove . . . quondam.

In *Much Ado about Nothing*, Margaret and Benedick exchange sexy banter:

> *Give us the swords; we have bucklers of our own.*
> *If you use them, Margaret, you must put in the*
> *pikes with a vice; and they are dangerous weapons for maids.*

Then Benedick mentions "a whole bookful of these quondam carpet-mongers, whose names yet run smoothly in the even road of a blank verse . . . were never so truly turned over and over as my poor self in love . . ."

Shakespeare—who better to leave a lexical condom conundrum than the Bard himself?

THE ENGLISH PARLIAMENT—
POETIC CENSURE OF THE QUONDAM

By the first decade of the eighteenth century, English jurors, poets, writers, and pundits were openly discussing and parodying the condom, confirming not only its common use but also its controversial place in the sexual lives of many Britons.

In 1708, as he stood at the dais before a packed Parliament, John Campbell, the Second Duke of Argyll, waved a *cundum* high over his head so that his fellow members could get a good look at it. As he flapped away, the agitated duke roared this description of the dreaded instrument: "Certaine instrument called a Quondam, occasioned ye debauching of a great number of Ladies of qualitie, and young gentlewomen."

This first mention of the condom (with the chronicler's interesting Scottish, or Shakespearean, spelling) in the Houses of Parliament shocked the conservative member of Parliament's audience, more for its theatrics than for the public display of the little linen sheath with its pink ribbon. But the duke, who was known as a "sober, thoughtful, a good husband . . . whose loftiness of mind did not prevent his harbouring the most illiberal contempt of women," was so offended by the increased use and increased public availability of the quondam that he was willing to make a fool of himself for the cause; he fervently hoped to make it a public offense to sell or use them.

Contrary to what he had hoped, Campbell's eccentric display did nothing but give his political detractors a rich opportunity to parody him, not because they were particularly defensive of the *device*, but because they hated the duke. He was a *Scottish* duke, but he was dedicated to the union of England and Scotland. Since his was the minority view among the Scottish members of Parliament, they took great pleasure in penning a little ditty for their condom-hating countryman.

In a brief verse, which referred to the condom as a disease preventative, Scottish Lord Belhaven wrote,

In a Scot's Answer to a British Vision

When Reasoning's answer'd
By seconded Votes
And speeches are banter'd
By outfield turn-coats
The Syringe* and Condum
Come both in request
While Virtuous Quondam
Is treated in Jest.

RHYME AND REASON, CHAPTER AND VERSE

Written in 1708, a longer, less politically driven bit of prose by an anonymous author also extolled the disease-preventing virtues of the condom. In the oddly named *Almonds for Parrots: With a Word or Two to a Scurrilous Satyr, Call'd, St. James' Park: With a Word or Two in Praise of Condons*, the author parodies the "happy invention" made of "gut," which "quench'd the heat of Venus's Fire and yet preserv'd the Flame of Love's Desire."

O matchless condon! thou'st secur'd thy Fame
To last as long as Condon is a Name.
Such mighty things are by they Influence done,
Thou ha'st the formost of this Age out-run.
Vulcan himself has been out-stript by thees,
Thou patron of the Paphian Deity.
For Mars's Heroes, shinn Arms he made;
But thou for Venus, takes up Vulcan's Trade.
Superior much, thou do'st the God out-shine.
Achilles Armour cannot match with thine.
Thine makes the Knight invulnerable still;
Condon has quench'd the heat of Venus's Fire,

---

*Syringe refers to the device used by many doctors and quacks to *cure* venereal disease.

And yet preserv'd the Flame of Love's Desire.

    O condon! bless'd must be thy teeming Brain
That proves at lenghth, Nature made nought in vain
But such capacious Heads as thine, can find
For what they were at first by her design'd.
Long had the Paeans of the Age, who shine
    In Arts, and boast themselves of Race divine;
Long had these Aeschulapian Heroes vex'd
Their leisure thoughts, and long their Minds perplex'd,
To search the Cause why Nature had assign'd
To Men and Brutes, a Gut the Learn'd call Blind;
Till Condon for the Great Invasion fam'd
Found out its use, and after him 'twas namd.
Hail! mighty Leader of the Condon Crew,
Who charge the Fair, arm'd Cap-a-pee, like you!
    To noble A-le first you did impart
The secret Knowledge of your saving Art:
Which, had you taught O/r/r/e/ry before.
ou'd sav'd his Calfs, not such as Israel did adore.
But such as he has offer'd to his Whore.
And now, who have we Illustrioius Race,
From my Lord's Valet, to his very Grace,
That can be said to be instructed right.
Unless he knows with Condons how to fight?
    Happy Invention! that is grown a Trade,
Whereby some Honest People get their Bread,
But they in ev'ry Market can't be had,
The Huckster-Dealers only will them sell,
at th'Park, Spring-Garden, Play-House or the Mall.
'Tis pitty that a Grant is not obtain'd.
that something may be to the Publick gain'd;
That like New Rome, New Britain may appear,
And our wise Laws appoint a Register
To enter Condon-Hawkers ev'ry Year.

A RAMBLE IN ST. JAMES'S PARK

Opened to the public by Charles II, by the eighteenth century St. James's Park had become an open-air den of iniquity. During the day, it was a place of assignation for adulterers and young people who were not supposed to be out alone together. At night, it was a haven for men on the make, prostitutes, homosexual liaisons, and every other kind of sexual encounter one can think of. It is here that many of the wondering condom sellers found a great market. It was so notorious, in fact, that Lord Rochester—a sexual rogue himself— penned this poem about the promiscuous park:

> *Nightly now beneath the trees' shade*
> *Are buggeries, rapes and incests made*
> *Unto this all-sin-sheltering Grove*
> *Whores of the Bulk and the Alcove*
> *Great Ladies, chamber maydes and Drudges,*
> *The Ragg Picker, and Heiress Trudges,*
> *Carmen, Divines, Great Lords, and Taylors,*
> *Prentices, Poets, Pimps and Gaolers,*
> *Footmen, Fine Fopps, do here arrive*
> *And here promiscuously they swive.*

At first read, it might seem odd that anyone would spend time penning prose about condoms, but this is really poking fun at the busy sex trade of that century. Stylewise, in spite of its lewd subject matter, it is reflective of eighteenth-century poetic verse and borrows both content and plenty of style from popular works, including Shakespeare's *Venus*. It also offers an amazing amount of information about condom use and sales in eighteenth-century London.

The mention of registering *Condon-Hawkers* helps to document the fact that condom peddlers were a common site throughout London, especially in places

THE GAY SHEATH

There is some controversy over when and why gay men began to use condoms: though most experts on the subject say that they were not used by gay men until the 1950s, and then only as a sex toy, poetry going back hundreds of years may offer clues to the contrary. There were likely gay men who knew or assumed that homosexual sex was just as likely to carry the threat of disease as a heterosexual liaison.

like St. James's Park, Spring Garden, and the Pall Mall, all spots popular with Londoners for their beauty and history, and well known as locations for illicit assignations between men and women, prostitutes and their customers—perfect locations, in other words, for selling sex aids.

There were actually two versions of *Almonds for Parrots* distributed around London, and in the unexpurgated version, there is also a glimpse into alternative lifestyles of the time. Although it began as a satire about sex for sale, *Almonds* also referred to the fact that places like St. James's Park were infamous locations for the homosexual rendezvous, and hinted at condom use by gay men:

> *But Art surpasses Nature; and we find*
> *Men may be transform'd into Woman-kind.*
> *O happy Change! But far more wond'rous Skill!*
> *That curse's Love's Wounds, without the Doctor's Pill:*
> *Anticipates ev'n Condon's secret Art,*
> *At first invented to secure the Part.*

UNLIKELY SONNETEERS

In his 1728 poem, *A Tale*, poet William Pattison offered an accurate description of what a condom of the day looked like: the "interceptive Shield" was colored a "dirty yellow and bound with blue." He also reminded his readers that the major difference between the cloth and the gut condom was that the gut variety worked best when wet . . . and that it smelled!

> *Of Parent Wave, from whence it came,*
> *Still mindful, the Italian Dame**
> *Ordains it shall all Sizes fit,*
> *Provided that it first be wet;*
> *And when put off to End of Time,*
> *Should smell of Fish and feel of Slime.*

---

*A reference to the goddess Aphrodite.

Even the English poet laureate Nicholas Rowe wrote of the *armour* that was gaining such favor in eighteenth-century England and Europe:

> *The Man, Dear Friend, who wears a condum,*
> *May scour the Hundreds round at random;*
> *Whether it please him to disport,*
> *In Wild-Street, or in Coulson's-Court;*
> *He fears no Danger from the Doxies,*
> *Laughs at their F????*, and scorns their Poxes.*

Another curious literary consideration of the condom was authored by the creatively named Roger Pheuquewell, Esq, who wrote *A New Description of Merryland*, an examination of the female anatomy thinly disguised as a travelogue. Mr. Pheuquewell told men that in order to protect themselves from Merryland's "dangerous Heat of the Climate" they had to put on "proper Cloathing . . . made of an extraordinary fine thin Substance, and contrived so as to be all of one Piece, and without a Seam, only about the Bottom it is generally bound round with a Scarlet Ribbon for Ornament."

> ## POETIC BURIALS
> *The poet laureate shared something else in common with his beloved Shakespeare; when Nicholas Rowe died in 1742, a monument in his honor was erected in the South Cross of Westminster Abbey, next to the Bard. It may be a good thing that visitors to the abbey are unaware of the "what else" these famous men shared in common.*

Mr. Pheuquewell apparently understood the beauty of seamless "cloathing"; for many centuries one of the biggest complaints about condom use came from women who hated being rubbed raw by a poorly fashioned seam.

THE GALLANT FRENCH

Not long after the publication of *Merryland* bespoke of the wonders of cloathing, another anonymous Frenchman published a detailed description

---

*F???? is left to the reader's imagination.

of the use of condoms among his fellow countrymen. Similar to earlier French works of fiction, *Histoire Amoureuse & Badine du Congres & de la Ville d'Utrecht*, printed in 1714, praised the virtues of the miraculous preventative that did not "interfere at all with pleasure." This excellent *armour*, raved Anonymous, was made of a very fine fabric or animal bladder, and was more effective than "if made from iron." His *armour* was to be fitted on the man's *gallant* only when he was ready to "thrust forward." Oh, and the *armour* was tied onto the man's *gallant* with a nice little ribbon.

A condom-loving Frenchman, one who was anything but anonymous, was famous in the aristocratic world of prerevolutionary France as an art critic and a social analyst. Louis Petit de Bachaumont was also passionate about the use of condoms.

A minor aristocrat himself, Bachaumont had access to the Parisian salons of that city's most influential eighteenth-century elite; there, he collected and chronicled in his personal journals the secrets of the rich and famous. To the horror of many, Bachaumont published the enormous collection of his diaries as *Memoires secrets de la republique des lettres* (Secret memories of the republic of letters). Although his writings were little more than spicy gossip, touted by the publisher as offering up all the details of "vaudevilles sur la cour" (circuses of romance), they were also an authentic reflection of the sexy, spirited, social, and sometimes debauched period of that era in French history.

Bachaumont specialized in discussing gossip and other people's sex lives, but he was serious when he recorded in his personal diary a couplet he had penned for a beautiful former ballerina: "You know the use of the condom. The condom, my daughter, is the law and the prophet." The quixotic verse illustrates the author's commitment to the little device as disease preventative and probably birth control, and his desire to pass on the wisdom of its use. It was also timely advice for the poor woman, who had had to turn to prostitution after her career in the ballet had ended badly.

HISTORY'S MOST PROTRACTED PROPHYLACTIC POETRY

The longest poetic work about con-doms, written around 1723 by an Anglican rector, White Kennett, has to be the *Ode to the Condom.* The son of the Bishop of Peterborough, Kennett praised the condom as birth control and disease preventative, rescuing women from "big Belly," and "the squawling Brat," as well as providing

> ## A CONDOM EULOGY
> *The* Oxford English Dictionary *defines* panegyrick *as a "public speech or published text in praise of a person or thing; a laudatory discourse; a eulogy, an encomium"—or—"a person who writes or delivers a eulogy or encomium." Was White Kennett praising or mourning his cundums?*

protection from "the Bubos." Neither the Church of England nor the bishop recorded for history any responses to this clergyman's prurient prose.

Ode to the Condom—A Panegyrick upon Cundum

> *O all ye Nymphs, in lawless Love's Disport*
> *Assiduous! whose ever open Arms*
> *Both Day and Night stand ready to receive*
> *The fierce Assaults of Britain's am'rous Sons!*
> *Whether with Golden Watch, or stiff Brocade*
> *You shine in Playhouse or the Drawing-room.*
> *Whores thrice magnificent! Delight of Kings,*
> *And Lords of goodliest Note; or in mean Stuffs*
> *Ply ev'ry Evening near St. Clement's Pile,*
> *Or Church of fam'd St. Dunstan, or in Lane,*
> *Or Alley's dark Recess, or open Street,*
> *Known by white Apron, bart'ring Love with Cit,*
> *Or strolling Lawyer's Clerk at cheapest Rate;*
> *Whether of Needham's or of Jordan's Train,*
> *Hear, and attend: In Cundum's mighty Praise*
> *I sing, for sure 'tis worthy of a Song.*
> *Venus, assist my Lays, thou who presid'st*
> *In City Ball or Courtly Masquerade,*

Goddess supreme! sole Authoress of our Loves
Pure and impure! whose Province 'tis to rule
Not only o'er the chaster Marriage Bed,
But filthiest Stews, and Houses of kept Dames!
To thee I call, and with a friendly Voice,
Cundum I sing—by Cundum now I cure
Boldly the willing Maid, by Fear a while
Kept virtuous, owns thy Pow'r, and takes thy Joys
Tumultuous; Joys untasted but by them.
Unknown big Belly, and squawling Brat,
Best Guard of Modesty! She riots now
Thy Vo'try, in the Fulness of thy Bliss."
Happy the Man, who in his Pocket keeps,
Whether with green or scarlet Ribband bound,
A well made Cundum—He, nor dreads the Ills
Of Shankers or Cordee, or Bubos dire!
"Thrice happy he—(for when in lewd Embrace
Of Transport-feigning Whore, Creature obscene!
The cold insipid Purchase of a Crown!
Bless'd Chance! Sight seldom seen! and mostly given
By Templar or Oxonian—Best Support
Of Drury and her starv'd Inhabitants;)
With Cundum arm'd he wagest am'rous Fight
Fearless, secure; nor Thought of future Pains,
Resembling Prick of Pins and Needle's Point,
E'er checks his Raptures, or disturbs his Joys!
So Ajax, Grecian Chief, with Seven-fold Shield,
Enormous! brav'd the Trojan's fiercest Rage;
While the hot daring Youth, whose giddy Lust
Or Taste too exquisite, in Danger's Spite
Resolves upon Fruition, unimpair'd
By intervening Armour, Cundum hight!
Scarce three Days past, bewails the dear-bought Bliss!
For now tormenting Sore with scalding Heat
Of Urine, dread Fore-runner of a Clap!

With Eye repentant, he surveys his Shirt,
Diversify'd with Spots of yellow Hue,
Sad Symptom of ten thousand Woes to come!
Now no Relief but from the Surgeon's Hand,
Or Pill-prescribing Leach, tremendous Sight
To Youth diseas'd! In Garret high he moans
His wretched Fate, where vex'd with nauseous Draughts
And more afflicting bolus, he, in Pangs
Unfelt before, curses the dire Results
Of lawless Revelling; from Morn to Eve
By never-casing keen Emeticks urg'd;
Nor slights he now his Grannum's sage Advice:
Nor feels he only but in megrim'd Head,
Head frought with Horror—Child of sallow Spleen,
Millions of idle Whims and Fancies dance
Alternate, and perplex his labouring Mind.
What erst he has been told of sad Mischance,
Either in Pox or Clap, of falling Nose,
Scrap'd Shins, and Buboes' Pains of vile Effect!
All feels the Youth, or fancies that he feels,
Nay, be it but a Gleet, or gentlest Clap,
His ill forboding Fears deny him Rest,
And fancied Poxes vex his tortur'd Bones;
Too late convinc'd of Cundum's sov'reign Use,
Hail Manes of Love-propagating Pimp!
Long since deceas'd, and long by me ador'd;
& gt; From whose prolific Brain, by lucky Hit,
Or Inspiration from all gracious Heaven,
First sprang the mighty Secret; Secret to guard
& gt; From Poison virulent of unsound Dame.
Hail, happy Albion, in whose fruitful Land
The wond'rous Pimp arose, from whose strange Skill
In inmost Nature thou hast reap'd more Fame,
More solid Glory, than from Newton's Toil;
Newton who next is England's noblest Boast:

If aught I can presage, as Smyrna once,
Chios and Colophon, and Rhodian Isle,
Famous for vast Colosos; and Argos fair
And Salamis, well known for Grecian Flight
with mighty Xerxes; and the Source of Arts,
High Athens! long contended for the Praise
Of Homer's Birth-place, egregious Bard!
In after Times so shall with warm Dispute
Europa's rival Cities proudly strive,
Ambitious each of being deem'd the Seat
Where Cundums first drew vital Air,
Too cruel Fate—Partial to human Race—
To us propitious—But O hard Decree!
Why, why so long in darksome Womb of Night
Dwelt the profound Arcanum, late reveal'd;
Say I not rather why, ye niggard Stars,
Are not your Blessings given unpall'd with Ill,
And Love, your greatest Blessing, free from Curse,
Curse of Disease! How many gallant Youths
Have fallen by the Iron Hand of Death
Untimely, immature: As if, to Love,
Your everlasting Purpose, were a Crime.
But, O ye Youths, born under happier Stars,
Britainnia's chiefest Hope! upon whose Cheeks
Gay Health sits smiling, and whose nervous Limbs
Sweet Ease, her Offspring fair! invigorates,
Unbrac'd as yet by foul Contagion,
Fav'rites of Fortune! let th' unhappy Lot
Of others teach you timely to beware;
That when replete with Love, and spur'd by Lust,
You seek the Fair-one in her Cobweb Haunts,
Or when allur'd by Touch of passing Wench,
Or caught by Smile insidious of the Nymph
Who in Green Box at Playhouse nightly flaunts,
And fondly calls thee to Love's luscious Feast,

> *Be cautious, stay a while 'till fitly arm'd*
> *With Cundum Shield, at Rummer best supply'd,*
> *Or never-failing Rose; so you may thrum*
> *Th' ecstatic Harlot, and each joyous Night*
> *Crown with fresh Raptures; 'till at least unhurt,*
> *And sated with the Banquet, you retire.*
> *By me forwarn'd thus may you ever treat*
> *Love's pleasing Paths in blest Security.*

FIVE

medical arguments against armour and a case of caveat emptor

DOCTORS, DEBATES, DEBAUCHEES, AND THE MRS. P'S

*I*n the seventeenth and eighteenth centuries, science and medicine had made a few modest gains. The circulation of the blood was understood, and many of the herbal potions coming from the Orient did actually have some healing qualities. Because this was an "age of war," some Western advances in treatment were made if only because of the many wounded soldiers who provided lots of practice. For instance, a French field surgeon decided, rightly so, that the standard practice of pouring boiling oil on an open wound was not productive. Instead, he suggested a poultice of egg, oil of rose, and turpentine, which was somewhat less painful and also had soothing and antiseptic qualities. That said, this was still not a good time to be sick.

There was, of course, no germ theory, so even though suturing was a positive new development in medicine, the needles used were rarely if ever washed. When the plague broke out in London in 1665, "miasmas" coming from sewers and cesspits were blamed, with few suspecting that personal cleanliness, or lack thereof, was actually the culprit. Chopping off limbs was still the most likely way to deal with crushed arms or legs and cases of gangrene, and doctors still thought the horn of a unicorn (where they found this necessary ingredient is a bit of a mystery) was an important healing agent, along with spiders' webs and powders made from the skulls of criminals.

Of course, there was the miraculous new drug also from China. Opium at least helped to make the pain go away, even if it did not cure any ills.

CUM HASTIS

So in an era of medical history when doctors were likely to answer the call to heal with a jolly good bleeding, when the notion of washing one's hands prior to moving from sick bed to child bed was not a consideration, and when barbers and quacks—whose credentials do not appear to be much different from *real* doctors—practiced medicine freely (and the average woman could hope to live to the ripe old age of forty), it is perhaps surprising that a handful of influential physicians spent a great deal of time and effort to publicly denounce the humble little condom. But they did just that.

In 1717, the physician sometimes referred to as England's first dermatologist and famous even in his own time as a surgeon, medical theorist, and author, Daniel Turner ranted against their increasing popularity. He condemned all use of the *condum* as "the best, if not the only Preservative our Libertines have found out at present; and yet, by reason of its blunting the Sensation, I have heard some of them acknowledge, that they had often chose to risqué a Clap, rather [than] engage *cum Hastis sic clypeatis* [with spears thus sheathed]."

Turner's contempt for the *preservative* was based on medical rather than moral grounds, and likely stemmed from his work with syphilis patients. The idea that a little piece of cloth or gut offered full immunity and protection from such an awful disease was, according to Turner, completely ridiculous. This is a notion that would haunt the little device many centuries later. Turner's diatribe against the condom may be logical in some ways, but it is difficult to understand just why he felt compelled to mention its "numbing" qualities: since this is unrelated to any medical concerns, perhaps he was worried about the *blunting of sensation*, believing that men would be seduced by the idea that it was an easy way to prevent disease, only to abandon it at the last minute because a *spear thus sheathed* could ruin the experience.

Jean Astruc, a French physician and contemporary of Turner's, and one of French king Louis XV's personal physicians, was an admirer of the English doctor's work on syphilis, and another anticondomite. In fact, Astruc was so impressed with Turner's writings condemning the condom that he wrote his own treatise, citing the other physician as the authority on the subject and quoting from that source.

Astruc's critique of the little bag made of "fine seamless animal bladders" poked fun at the Englishmen who foolishly used this objectionable little device, falsely believing it would keep them safe from their own "debauched" behaviors. Well known in France for his own work on syphilis, it seems that Astruc was not aware of the fact, or was unwilling to admit, that the condom was as popular in France as it was in England. In 1736 he wrote:

> I hear from the lowest debauchees who chase without restraint after the love of prostitutes, that there are recently employed in England skins made from soft and seamless hides in the shape of a sheath, and called condoms in English, with which those about to have intercourse wrap their penis as in a coat of mail in order to render themselves safe in the dangers of an ever doubtful battle. They claim, I suppose, that thus mailed and with spears sheathed in this way, they can undergo with impunity the chances of promiscuous intercourse. But in truth they are greatly mistaken.
>
> They ought to arm their penises with oak, guarded with a triple plate of brass, instead of trusting to a thin bladder, who are fond of committing a part so capable of receiving infection to the filthy gulph of a Harlot. Surely it is far better to live chastely, or to partake the pleasures of venery with permission and safety, than to make use of so filthy and nasty an invention.

Astruc's acerbically witty comments are proof that by the eighteenth century the French were convinced that the sheath had been invented by the English. In fact, by the early 1700s, the French routinely referred to it as the *Anglaise d'redincoat, redingotes d'Anglaise,* and the *redingotes d'Angleterre* (the English raincoat) or *la capote Anglaise* (the English cape). Curiously, the English returned the favor and frequently referred to theirs as the *baudruche,* or the French letter—a euphemism still in use today.

Although he was certainly out of touch with the French sexual mores of the day, Astruc does address one of the genuine problems with the condoms of old—and not so old. Besides a complete lack of understanding about germs and the need for personal hygiene—the average eighteenth-century European might have chosen to bathe once a year, or *not*—condoms had to be made individually, by hand, and could be expensive, ranging from a few pennies to a few schillings or francs each (roughly one to five pounds or dollars in twenty-first-century terms), so men often reused them, especially the linen variety. Laundering their sheaths, on the other hand, was a haphazard process. Although there is no way to know just how reuse might or might not have contributed to the actual spread of venereal disease, Astruc (and Turner) may actually have associated the condom with contagion rather than prevention. A more likely explanation, though, is that condoms made of animal intestines were often riddled with tiny holes, rendering them useless. And even with the nice silk ribbons attached, they could fall off if used too vigorously.

HISTORIC LEXICON

Historically speaking the condom has had a lot of noms de plume: baudruche, condum, condum, quandum, quandon, English raincoat, Anglaise d'redincoat, rubber, night cap, sheath, armour, codpiece, un petit linge, conton, instrument, proper Cloathing, interceptive shield, preservative, French letter, letter, overcoat, coat, device, filthy slipper, machinery, cundum, dead letter, redingotes d'Anglaise, skin, bladder, machine, redingotes d'Angleterre, preventative bag, raincoat, capote, Cytherean shield, Gant des dames, Colotte d'assurance, Peau divine, Chemisette, Posthocalyptrons, Cutherean Shield, assurance cap, and un petit sac de peau de Venise.

Other criticisms by Europe's anticondom physicians appeared somewhat later in the century. These were not, however, concerned with the condom's connection to disease prevention; rather, they were against the little item because of its use—frequently mentioned in eighteenth-century literature—as a birth control device.

In 1750, English doctor Thomas Short blasted the "nefarious Practices used by wicked Wretches to prevent Conception from their carnal Gratification." Although Short railed against all methods of birth control, the condom was apparently enough of a threat to the moral health of the nation that it always featured in his lambastes.

Later, in 1767, the same Dr. Short was still complaining about "so many wicked Arts . . . daily used to prevent Conception" and by the use of "Instruments . . . to prevent Conception." The law, Dr. Short felt, "should make sure that the instrument maker be . . . punished or hanged with the Criminals. . . . There can be little doubt that a medical man would be aware of the . . . condom, and that these are here being condemned." Lord Campbell would have been proud.

THE STORY OF A SELF-PORTRAIT

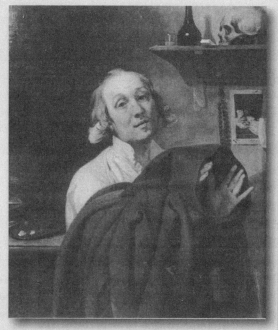

German artist Johan Zoffany was a popular artist of the eighteenth century well known for his homoerotic themes, as well as his more traditional presentations. He was said to have been quite a social climber and counted among his friends and acquaintances Captain Cook—with whom Zoffany was supposed to have sailed on his second voyage, only to cancel at the last moment—and the empress Maria Theresa.

The artist painted for a number of royals around Europe, including the British, and much of his work is displayed today in Florence's Uffizi Gallery and the Galleria Nazionale in Parma; this includes his Self-Portrait. The work is perhaps his most unique since Zoffany dressed in a Franciscan habit, and painted condoms hanging right behind him; experts have interpreted the work to be the artist's attempt to create a visual juxtaposition between love and the restrictions imposed by "religiosity." One art critic described Zoffany's theme as "confronted with one's mortality, religious piety again triumphs over sexual license." Maybe or maybe not, but it proved that the artist understood the value of washing his sheaths.

EUROPEAN VARIATIONS ON A THEME

In the early 1830s, the German physician Friedrich Adolph Wilde wrote about the use of condoms, both the male and the female varieties. His only concern about the male condom was that those he experimented with were not of particularly high quality and tended to break (he did not know about Casanova's little party trick). This led Wilde to recommend them with some reluctance, and to assure his readers that the female condom—a rubber cap or pessary—was superior because it was safer.

Another German doctor who advocated birth control insisted that the poor should have small families. His condom was actually infibulation, *that particularly painful and gross procedure identical to the Roman model of more than a thousand years prior. Actually, as with the Romans who advocated this procedure, the real intent behind infibulation was actually to discourage the wearer from having sex at all, a sort of surgical abstinence.*

This German physician was quite the eccentric; determined he had found the cure to overpopulation, he even proposed a state-sponsored infibulation program that included policing the men who had had the procedure. Along with drafting directions on how to infibulate *so that any physician could perform the procedure, the good doctor also made up a roster of punishments for wrongdoers caught cheating.*

German writer, researcher, and physician Christoph Girtanner is the only well-known medical expert from the time to castigate the condom from both angles—as disease preventative *and* as birth control. He also made it clear that condoms were an *English* (not a German or even a French) invention and that he considered them something only "debauchees" (an apparently universal pejorative for anyone using condoms) would ever use. In his 1788 book, *Abhandlung uber die Venerische Krankheit* (Treatise about the Venereal Disease), Girtanner, who had also been influenced by Astruc's work, described the methods the dreadful debauchees used to protect themselves:

> It is necessary in the meanwhile that I cite once more one of these means, because today it is considered a current custom and considered infallible by the debauchees who go to excess. On this occasion I proved, as I have proved in other passages in this work, how difficult it is to speak on the

subject which can be of interest to the human race and at the same time guard against offending modesty. The German language appears too chaste to furnish decent words on subjects so shameful.

Meanwhile the matter is too important to allow it to pass in silence. I wish to speak of the fish membranes which serve to protect the man's member during copulation. This shameful invention which suppresses and annihilates completely the only natural end of cohabitation, namely procreation, comes from England, where these instruments were used for the first time under the debauched reign of Charles II. Even today they bear the name of their inventor; they diminish pleasure and annihilate the natural end of cohabitation; finally they are insufficient to assure immunity, for the least hole will permit contagion. And again it may happen that during coitus the membrane may tear by a strong strain.

TOBIAS SMOLLET

Printed in 1748, Smollet's popular book Roderick Random *described what happened to eighteenth-century prostitutes when they contracted syphilis, surely enough to make the good doctors rethink their rabid anti-condom stance:*

The most fashionable woman of the towns is as liable to contagion as one in a much humbler sphere; she infects her admirers, her situation is public; she is avoided, neglected, unable to support her usual appearance, which however, she strives to maintain as long as possible; her credit fails, she is obliged to retrench, and become a night walker; her malady gains ground, she tampers with her constitution, and ruins it; her complexion fades, she grows nauseous to every dog, finds herself reduced to a starving condition, is tempted to pick pockets, is detected, committed to Newgate, where she remains in a miserable condition, till she is discharged because the plaintiff will not appear to prosecute her. Nobody will afford her lodgings, the symptoms of her distemper are grown outrageous, she sues to be admitted into an hospital, where she is cured at the expense of her nose; she is turned out into the streets, depends upon the addresses of the lowest class, is fain to allay the rage of hunger and cold with gin, degenerates into a brutal insensibility, rots and dies upon a dunghill.

THE SINFUL MACHINE

Others spoke out against the condom, but with even greater vehemence and with a distinctly religious edge. One author believed the condom simply encouraged men to go forth and behave in a sinful manner, claiming the device should have been illegal in a "Christian Country." He also berated anyone who advised men to "use Machinery, and to fight in Armour," or tried to get others to participate in "a practice which promoted wicked, sinful behavior." And anyone who used it for birth control? That was wrong because it was akin to masturbation—also a major sin.

Girtanner pretty much covers it all: the incorrect history of the condom, its origins so impure that the *chaste* German language just did not offer the vocabulary to describe the evils of the *membrane*, and his apparent assumptions—or personal experiences—about how they *diminish pleasure* (another universal belief among the anticondom medical experts).

In spite of his hatred of the device, the German doctor was an avid traveler and inadvertently helped to chronicle its widespread use and availability throughout Europe. He reported seeing them peddled in cities, in open-air markets, taverns, and other "retail" outlets in Russia, England, his native Germany, and France—more confirmation of their incredible popularity. Like his English counterpart, Dr. Short, Girtanner was also shocked and amazed that the police in Moscow, St. Petersburg, Paris, London, and Berlin did not step in to arrest the condom peddlers in order to end the *obscene* open-market approach to condom sales: "The negligence of the police, who do not seek to prevent the sale of an invention so shameful and so detrimental to repopulation, is in truth, inconceivable."

By the eighteenth century, the condom had inspired a diverse group of men of letters, physicians, and even the clergy to express their opinions of the little device. These, however, were the opinions of an elite few, of men who considered themselves experts in not only human health (specifically syphilis) but in human behavior. What they failed to recognize or admit was that public opinion—and practice—was what drove the manufacture, sale, and use of condoms all over the Western world. They were not the first and they would not be the last to make that mistake.

For all the complaints and criticisms, the condom market continued to grow and thrive throughout the eighteenth century. But who was actually meeting the demand, producing and selling to an ever-expanding market? And why would anyone decide upon such an odd profession? The simple answer is one that applied to the condom marketplace well into the twentieth century: an eclectic mix of entrepreneurs, down-and-outs, intellectuals, eccentrics, and crooks.

THE UNHEALTHY SIDE OF SHEATH PRODUCTION

Condom production, though almost unchanged for many millennia, was by the seventeenth century quite a diversified industry; some operations managed to thrive with only one or two employees, others had trained staff, each with their own tasks to perform. The Mrs. P's would have had a staff of young women working in a sort of primitive assembly line, tucked away in the back rooms and basements of the ladies' shops. Making sheaths from linen was a simple enough job for anyone who could use a needle, and working with prepared gut was not terribly different, but the women (and some men) who refined those guts were not so lucky and probably had rather short careers in the cundum business.

Sulphur—sulfur—and lye were the principal ingredients in making the dried caeca into a usable, pliable fabric. Sulfur, especially when heated to such a degree that it permeated the gut, had terrible side effects and would have caused burning and irritation of the skin, gastrointestinal problems, dizziness, convulsions, muscle pain, eye burning (and blindness if the eyes were directly exposed), thirst (water was not potable and drinking ale or cider while working with these chemicals was not a good idea), and respiratory infections. Ditto lye. This made the production side of the business much more harrowing than just sewing together the finished products, with their little silk ribbons.

PROPHYLACTIC PRODUCTION

Animal intestines had been used as protection for centuries, if not millennia, before the *Classical Dictionary of the Vulgar Tongue* was first printed in London in 1783. Written by the aptly named Captain Francis Grose, the dictionary offered this *learned* definition:

> **Cundum,** *the dried gut of sheep, worn by men in the act of coition, to prevent venereal infection, said to have been invented by one Colonel Cundum . . .*

Although making a condom was not terribly difficult and had been mastered by peoples from many cultures over many centuries, it was something that had generally been done by individuals for personal use or by those who specialized in making just a few at a time for special clients. Large-scale production-for-profit did not begin in earnest until the late seventeenth century.

At that time, although many people continued to fabricate their own, entrepreneurs had discovered a nice little business niche, especially in the big cities of Europe. There, visiting men of wealth were likely to want protection while they savored the ready-sex of the big city. And residents who could afford the prefabricated variety were unlikely to want something as primitive as homemade *armour*.

Part of the appeal for manufacturers was that condoms could be produced in very small spaces, needing only a table or a workbench and a few basic supplies. Animal intestines, or guts, were cheap and readily available at any butcher shop or sausage supplier. The intestine of one sheep could make dozens of condoms, and the ribbon necessary to keep them in place could be purchased very inexpensively from any milliner or haberdasher.

Making linen condoms was more challenging, since they required careful stitching and were expected to be longer lasting than the gut variety. Many were also treated with chemical solutions (some no more than herbal oils and water, others more caustic, such as lye-based concoctions), intended as extra protection from disease but some of which also acted—accidentally—as spermicide. Although linen condoms were available through to the end of the eighteenth century, because they were more expensive to produce and to purchase and not as comfortable as gut, they had lost favor by the 1800s.

The method of production for making gut condoms remained the same for about three hundred years, well into the twentieth century: the intestinal material (caeca) was soaked in water for several hours, then macerated in a weak alkaline lye solution, which was changed every twelve hours: this was done over a one- to two-day period. Then the intestinal material was carefully scraped to remove the mucous membrane, using primitive metal instruments like cheap kitchen knives and long iron nails.

The chemicals and scraping left just the peritoneal and muscular coat of the intestine, which was exposed to the "vapour of burning brimstone"— a pot of sulfur, placed over an open flame until it let off a sulfuric steam that helped soften the gut. Finally, the softened sheet of what was left of the original intestine was washed in lye soap and water.

Oblong-shaped pieces of the gut were cut out with large, primitive shears, then small holes were cut or punched around the top edges. If the final consumer were lucky, the manufacturer might examine the pieces for tiny holes—a very rare occurrence judging by a French physician's note in 1770. He complained that his *redingotes d'Anglaise* were "riddled with a whole lot of pores." Finally, the still-wet strip was "bordered at the open end with a ribonad," ready for sale.

BAUDRUCHES FINES, SUPERFINES, SUPERSUPERFINES— GOOD, BETTER, BEST

By the early part of the eighteenth century, the condom's tremendous popularity had led to a demand for better, more comfortable models. Savvy entrepreneurs responded by diversifying their goods, offering a variety of qualities and sizes. Living up to their reputation as the inventors of the sheath, English manufacturers led the way in the effort to meet consumer demand—and they added a little extra panache by giving them fancy French names like *baudruches fines*, *superfines*, and *supersuperfines*, popular euphemisms for about two hundred years.

Even though manufacturers worked hard to produce a finer condom, the materials used and the methods of curing did not change. Intestines of sheep, cows, or lambs were prepared in the same manner as the one-size-fits-all model, but instead of just an oblong sack with a ribbon at the top, the fines were shaped and made smoother by being placed over oiled molds. These glass penis-shaped casts were sized small, medium, and large and were ordered from local glass blowers, men who must have had delightful senses of humor! By molding the gut, instead of a man tying a beribboned bag over his "yard" (the eighteenth-century man's favorite reference to his penis), the better-quality condom was nicely tailored and offered an improved fit.

Better yet, there were the *baudruches superfines*, which were made in the same manner as the *baudruches fines*, but the *superfines* were rubbed with oil scented with essences of flowers and spices (partly an effort to overcome the unpleasant smells that accompanied sex in a population that bathed very rarely, partly to make the chemically treated intestinal wall smell a bit less earthy), then rubbed with smooth glass to polish them.

And finally, there were the ultimate *baudruches superfines doubles*, which were actually two guts placed over one another while still moist, so that the "two insides adhere together." Although these were the pièce de résistance of all condoms, and doubling up on the carefully prepared fabric was intended to offer the ultimate protection, the *doubles* were actually not as popular as their lesser counterparts because they deadened sensation in a big way.

STINKY LONDON

Both public and private places smelled terrible in eighteenth-century London: rainwater full of animal waste and rotting debris blocked up drains, which overflowed into courtyards and side alleys. Ditches stunk of urine, rat droppings and rotting wood, filling the stairwells of poorly constructed apartments with their odors. Congealing blood from the butchers and slaughterhouses, and caustic lye scents filled the air near any tannery. Inside, damp featherbeds reeked, unwashed sheets let off their own perfume, and pungent chamber pots filled the air with a sickly sweet smell. And people . . . sweat and unwashed bodies, the horrors of rotting teeth, along with the breath of onions and intestinal parasites chewing up their innards, terrible— but the smell of eighteenth-century sex? That probably goes beyond mere words.

GLASSBLOWERS AND TOASTS

The glassblowers of Europe must have had excellent senses of humor. Not only did they fill every order for the bottles used to mold guts and later dip rubber, but some— specifically those in Scotland—were asked to "blow" an amazing drinking glass. At least one eighteenth-century men's club contracted to have "prick glasses" made; these unusual phallic vessels were intended not only for very particular celebrations, but also to double as dribble glasses. The unsuspecting toaster went to take a sip and ended up wearing his beverage of choice.

Interestingly, no matter the quality, price, or size, each condom was trimmed to a standard seven- or eight-inch length—and of course they all had pretty silk ribbons (pink, scarlet, and blue were the favored colors) fitted around the top, because no matter how nicely they were molded, even the fanciest *baudruche* still would not stay on without its little bow.

The problem with even the highest-quality gut condoms, though, was that no matter how much brimstoning and scented oils were employed, the material could rub tender parts the wrong way. And if the skins were not properly rinsed and soaked repeatedly in fresh water to remove all the chemicals, they could leave nasty burns and cause vaginal infections. With linen condoms, the seams could cause lesions. But for those who wanted the best of both worlds, sex and safety, *condoms, baudruches, armour, sheaths,* and *redingotes d'Anglaises* were worth the impediments. Their popularity grew throughout the ensuing centuries.

FROGGIE GOES A COURTIN'

In the late eighteenth century, Lazzaro Spallanzani, a professor of metaphysics and logic and self-styled scientist, taught and researched at three different Italian universities during his busy career. Fascinated by the role of semen in reproduction, Spallanzani sought to prove once and for all that it was a necessary "ingredient" in reproduction. Interestingly, the professor may not have been terribly well read on this issue or he would have realized that men all over the world were using condoms as birth control. Though it is very difficult to imagine how he did it, he claimed that to prove his theory, he covered the penises of frogs with linen sheaths; he later wrote that after the frogs had had congress no new frogs appeared.

THE MRS. P'S AND LONDON'S *MACHINE WARS*

Throughout Europe, condoms were bought and sold in a variety of locations, including pubs, barbershops, chemist shops, open-air markets, by street vendors, and at the theater. As evidenced by the prose of the time, London's St. James's Park, Spring-Garden, Bow Street, and the Pall Mall were known to be major outlets for outdoor condom sales. Men and women peddled them out-of-doors, from the baskets and bags they carried on their backs and on top of their heads, from pushcarts, or simply from their pockets.

This ragtag sales force was made up of out-of-work actors, down-and-out prostitutes, unsuccessful con men, as well as "legitimate" hawkers who saw a chance to diversify. They could be found selling their wares in all weathers, at all hours, and were such a common sight that condom sales became part of the local landscape. And the beauty of the business was that it was not as weather dependent as others like the fresh vegetable or the fruit market. In fact, the market really boomed during the winter, with most people housebound and looking for indoor entertainment. There were even complaints about some of the more aggressive condom salespeople, who when business was slow, were not shy about targeting men they thought looked like potential customers.

Because of their high visibility, there was a move to tax condom salespeople as legitimate peddlers, but the authorities dropped the idea because they did not want to be associated with the little item. The conservative lawmakers were fearful that by taxing this kind of business, they would be legitimizing it and it would be perceived by the public as putting a stamp of approval on illicit sex.

For more than 150 years, the issue of whether condom enterprise was a legitimate business, or not, came up repeatedly in Europe and later in the United States. It is doubtful anyone in the industry was troubled by lack of good standing, however. It simply meant greater profits, no strings attached.

> *Do as sage Ch-s-l-n is wont to do,*
> *For greater Safety put on two:*
> *With red Bag pendant on your Baws below.*
>
> Advice from a "cundum" manufacturer

LONDON'S CONDOM WARS

Although most hawkers of condoms were pretty colorful, none could match the dynamic—and certainly most public—condom purveyors in London: the feuding Mrs. P's.

The London Condom Wars began in the early eighteenth century, fought between three of the leading manufacturers of the little device. With an advertising blitz worthy of any modern American political campaign, Mrs. Mary Perkins and the two Mrs. Philipses began a public feud over who sold the best condoms.

The saga began in 1731 with the first Mrs. Philips, who started her retail business selling her homemade *machines* —yet another euphemism made popular in eighteenth-century London—in two of that city's most famous (and infamous) pubs, both popular watering holes since the time of the Stuarts. This first Mrs. P divided her time between The Rummer and The Grape and the Rose, peddling her wares to their colorful patrons, including London's Freemasons who conducted their secret meetings at these hostelries throughout the seventeenth and eighteenth centuries.

THE GRAPE AND THE ROSE

Mrs. Philips got her start at this busy watering hole, before going independent and opening up her own retail establishment. After she left, the owner found his own niche in the strange netherworld of London's sex industry.

John Harrison, whose nom de plum was Jack Harris, was the writer of a best-selling book, Harris' List of Covent Garden Ladies. The first edition came out in 1757, and remained in print for thirty years, being regularly updated. His writing earned the author the nickname "Pimp General to the People of England," basically because the book was considered a necessary tool for men who wanted a guide to the best, or most interesting, prostitutes in London. It is quite amazing, in fact, that this busy barkeep, an acquaintance of famous characters like James Boswell, had the time to explore and catalog in such detail the delights of places like Bow Street and Naked-Boy Court in the Strand. Mr. Harris also had a small side business in selling condoms to the same men who came to buy a copy of his little guide, which he claimed eventually sold more than 250,000 copies.

Mrs. Philips quickly became one of the most successful condom producers in England, perhaps even on the Continent, and opened her own wholesale/retail outlet, where a team of women produced all sorts of machines in a small room at the back of her shop. She did so well, making so much money selling condoms not only to individuals and local businesses but also to customers all over Europe, that Mrs. Philips decided to cash in on her success and retire. In 1766 she sold her business to Mrs. Mary

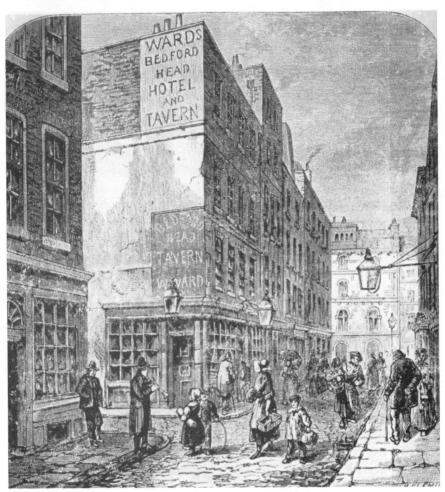

The Mses. Philipses' London

Perkins. By then, the first Mrs. P had been producing condoms at the "sign of the Green Canister on Half Moon Street" for more than thirty-five years.

After ten years of peaceful retirement, away from the daily grind of condom production and sales, Mrs. Philips reemerged, claiming she had heard a rumor about Mrs. Perkins. She said she had been told that this lady was not keeping to her high standards of manufacture. Mrs. Philips was so concerned about the bad news that she decided to go back to work. She opened a new condom business located at the "Orange Court at the sign of the Golden Fan and Rising Sun," near Leicester Fields.

Determined to regain her original market, and to get Mrs. Perkins's shoddy goods off the shelves, Mrs. Philips designed an admirable marketing blitz. She hired young men to hand out her handbills in crowded public streets and to distribute them to the most likely secondary retail outlets. The advertisements offered a range of "skins and bladders" to "apothecaries, chymists, druggiest &c." They also boasted about Mrs. Philips's select and diverse clientele, which she claimed included "ambassadors, foreigners, gentlemen and captains of ships, &c." who took advantage of the best deal "going abroad . . . with any quantity of the best goods in England, on the shortest notice and lowest price." Mrs. Philips was proud of the fact that she filled orders to be shipped to "France, Spain, Portugal, Italy, and other foreign places." But the best part of her marketing strategy was her actors who wandered the streets singing her very own jingle, extolling the virtues of her fine goods:

> *To guard yourself from shame or fear,*
> *Votaries to Venus, hasten here;*
> *None in our wares e'er found a flaw*
> *Self-preservation's nature's law.*

It was the wording of the returning Mrs. Philips's advertisements, publicly criticizing the quality of Mrs. Perkins's machines, that really started the war. Mrs. Philips stated in her sales campaign that she was forced to return to business because she had "been prevailed upon by her friends to reassume the same again upon representations that, since her declining, they cannot procure any goods comparable to those she used to vend."

The story became complicated when a second Mrs. Philips materialized and declared in circulars that the first Mrs. Philips was dead! The second Mrs. P turned out to be none other than Mrs. Perkins, angry over not just Mrs. Philips reappearing and competing for her business, but because of the direct knock at the quality of her goods.

The second Mrs. Philips, aka Mrs. Perkins, even put out her own handbills proclaiming "some evil-minded person has given out handbills, that

ENGLAND'S HAWKERS AND PEDDLERS
A contemporary account of a group of "traders" vying with the condom peddlers:

Through the busy concourse flowing up and down the thoroughfares from dawn to dusk, street-criers took their way, bearing wares upon their heads in wicker baskets, before them on broad trays, or slung upon their backs in goodly packs. And as they passed, their voices rose above the general din, calling "Fair lemons and oranges, oranges and citrons!" "Cherries, sweet cherries, ripe and red!" "New flounders and great plaice; buy my dish of great eels!" "Rosemary and sweet briar; who'll buy my lavender?" "Fresh cheese and cream!" "Lily-white vinegar!" "Dainty sausages!" which calls, being frequently intoned to staves of melody, fell with pleasant sounds upon the ear. [These hawkers so seriously interfered with legitimate traders that in 1694 they were forbidden to sell any goods or merchandise in any public place within the city or liberties, except in open markets and fairs, on penalty of forty shillings for each offence, both to buyers and sellers.] Moreover, to these divers sights and sounds were added ballad singers, who piped ditties upon topics of the day; quacks who sold nostrums and magic potions; dancers who performed on tight-ropes; wandering musicians; fire-eaters of great renown; exhibitors of dancing dolls, and such like itinerants "as make show of motions and strange sights," all of whom were obliged to have and to hold "a license in red and black letters, under the hand and seal of Thomas Killigrew, Esq., master of the revels to his sacred majesty Charles II."

the machine warehouse, the Green Canister, in Half-moon-street in the Strand, is removed, it is without foundation, and only to prejudice me, this being the old original shop, still continued by the successor of the late Mrs. Philips, where gentlemen's order shall be punctually observed in the best manner, as usual."

Mrs. Perkins, or the second Mrs. Philips, went so far as to steal the first Mrs. Philips's jingle, hiring her own troubadours to sing it while they distributed handbills advertising her wares—which included not only machines, but snuff, soap, essences, and "Ladie's black sticking plaister." The plaister was a popular item with women who cut out cute little hearts and stars to stick over small scars on their faces, a common and unfortunate result of smallpox.

Mrs. Perkins was far more diversified than the first Mrs. Philips, but that lady had a nationwide, even European-wide, wholesale business in machine sales, so presumably, although the final outcome of this public feud is unknown, the two Mrs. P's must have ended their battle and got on with the business of producing and selling condoms. Certainly, whatever happened at the close of the Condom Wars, few Londoners of the time would not have known about these ladies and their dueling machines.

REMEMBER TO RECYCLE

Although not directly involved in London's Condom Wars, perhaps the most colorful women who sold the little device were those who also saw treasures in other people's trash. Miss Jenny, for instance, was most famous for her excellent tavern, where she offered "extra" services to gentlemen in her upstairs rooms. She was also well known for her ample supply of good-quality condoms, many of which were surprisingly affordable. Unbeknownst to her customers, Miss Jenny's staff were very good about collecting them after they had been discarded, so that she could recycle them, which is why they were so cheap. Fortunately for the unsuspecting users of the slightly used machines, she did launder them before reuse.

And then there was Mrs. Jenkins, a madam who owned a brothel known to Londoners and visitors alike for catering to customers with kinky tastes. Mrs. Jenkins's "girls" were especially adept

RIBBONS AND BOWS

Although there were numerous materials used to make condoms, the common thread in production for many centuries was the little pink, scarlet, or blue silk ribbons woven around the opening of each, necessary to actually keep them on. But who were the ribbon makers?

They were second-wage earners, married to men who worked at seasonal or poorly paying jobs, or girls from poor families lucky enough not to end up as household servants or worse. Many of the women who produced the silk ribbons were employed in the East End of London, where the largest such manufacturer was located. This was an almost exclusively female-based industry— labor wise—and it was one of the few places the wives of sailors could find employment. Most ribbon was purchased by haberdashers, almost 40 percent of whom were also women. Both the business of making and selling ribbon and that of making and selling condoms were femalecentric and both offered regular employment, uninterrupted by the season—in fact, business boomed during the colder months, when demand soared.

at the practice of flagellation, which was eighteenth-century England's favorite sadomasochistic sexual ritual. She also ran an excellent side trade in the buying, washing, and reselling of "slightly used *baudruches*."

Other women purveyors of condoms in London, like Mother Lewis, seemed to have stayed away from the heated battles and the peculiar dealings of some of their fellow vendors, preferring to sell their wares in pubs and taverns. There was also yet another Mrs. Philips (with the interesting first name Con) who at least deserved the award for having been in the condom business the longest—she was still selling them from her shop on Bedford Street in the 1760s and had opened her business in 1701.

Elsewhere in Europe, business was also brisk, though less colorful than the battling Mrs. Philipses. Merchant Mathijs van Mordechay Cohen, one of Amsterdam's better-known eighteenth-century purveyors, did a brisk business in condoms, which he made himself from lambs' bladders and silk ribbons; the Russians, Germans, French, Swiss, and many others were also producing a variety of condoms for their own local markets, unmolested by taxes, legal restraints, customs, or duties.

RAGS, NUTS, AND YARDS

Condom salespeople may have inadvertently been given a marketing freebie from an odd source. Though not a manufacturer or salesman, in 1708 Englishman John Marten did get some attention for his part in promoting their use. A self-proclaimed scientific expert (more accurately referred to by medical historians as a "quack"), Marten actually promoted condom use as a cure for syphilis, advertising his "curative" in London newspapers.

Mr. Marten was not selling a cure-all condom, however. His advertisements claimed that he possessed a secret formula, a liquid the customer was supposed to dip his rag into, a sure cure for "the problem"—or better yet, it was best used prior to catching a disease in the first place.

In his advertisement for the liquid solution, Marten included his own sage advise about just how to get the most out of his formula:

Lint or Linen Rags be divers times wet in it, and dried in the Shade, of a sufficient bigness to involve the Glans or Nut of the Man's Yard, or to cover the inner parts of the Privity of the woman, and applied and kept on for a while before Engagement, will so harden the Members, dry up the superfluous Moistnesses, and resist Putrefaction, as that no one that uses them shall ever be afflicted with the Pox.

There are no records as to how well the formula sold, but Marten certainly had a way with words. And he was not alone in his colorful language describing condoms, condom use, and the excellent reasons for employing them. Besides the faceless Freemasons, Mrs. Jenkins's odd clients, and "ambassadors, foreigners, gentlemen and captains of ships," some of history's most famous, and infamous, men truly loved their *machines, armour,* and *redingotes d'Anglaise.*

SIX

the most famous, and infamous, users of all

THE CELEBRITY OVERCOAT

By this Machine secure, the willing Maid
Can taste Love's Joys, nor is she more afraid
Her swelling Belly should, or squalling Brat,
Betray the Luscious Pastime she has been at.

The Machine, 1744

The eighteenth century brought forth some of the most profound political and philosophical changes so far experienced in Western history. New nations were formed and the first modern democracies were born. Mozart and Handel composed some of the most beautiful, complex music heretofore heard, and Captain Cook discovered the fantastic Pacific Islands. But while Voltaire and Rousseau argued over lofty issues like education, democracy, and religion, and Hume, Paine, and Bentham explored the concepts that would eventually give shape and form to coming cultural explorations and conflicts, other famous and infamous men of the Enlightenment were exploring somewhat earthier topics.

In fact, the Enlightenment's most exalted lovers held their humble little condoms in very high regard. In their letters, diaries, and memoirs, these men sang the praises of their *armour*, *machines*, and *redingotes d'Anglaise*. And all spoke of their little sheaths with affection.

One of these men is often referred to as the world's greatest lover.

Claiming to have come from a minor aristocratic family—he *could* boast a great-grandfather who had sailed with Christopher Columbus—Giacomo Girolamo Casanova was actually the son of two Venetian actors from whom he probably inherited his larger-than-life presence. Casanova lived a checkered but very colorful existence, full of misadventure, free sex, multiple prison stays, and lots of near misses. He was a gambler, with women and in business, which made him a very rich (and sometimes a very poor) man. When he was in the money, he frequently socialized with some of the most eminent leaders of his time. And his prowess as a lover became so well known that modern English uses his name as a synonym for "sexual rogue."

But Casanova displayed an unusually practical side for a man who slept with women all over Europe: he used condoms. His principal reason for doing so was to avoid the *complications* likely when sleeping with other men's wives, but it was mostly to prevent infection.

In his *Histoire de Ma Vie* (History of My Life) written around 1789, Casanova mentions his "redingotes d'Angleterre," or *English raincoats*. In spite of the fact that he had earned his letters in canon and civil law at the University of Padua, he was obviously unaware that a fellow Italian had popularized the early modern Western condom. Like so many other Europeans, Casanova thought they had originated in England, calling them the "little preventive bag invented by the English to save the fair sex from anxiety." He described his as "a little coat of very fine and transparent skin, eight inches long and closed at one end, with a narrow pink ribbon slotted through the open end" and an "overcoat that puts one's mind at rest . . . wonderful preventive against an accident which might lead to frightful repentance."

Casanova also used his bag as a part of foreplay, innocently requesting his partner's assistance in putting it on. He even invented the party trick of entertaining ladies by blowing up his raincoats like balloons—which was also a good way to ensure they did not have any tiny holes in them.

Perhaps surprisingly—he was the first to brag about how women fell all over themselves as they sought his sexual favors, and how easily he was able to get them "to bed"—one of Casanova's more colorful condom experiences took place in a brothel. On this presumably rare visit to a prostitute, he had forgotten his overcoat. When he asked the madam for one, she tried to sell him an inferior variety that was far too coarse for his aristocratic member, and he demanded better quality. The madam offered to sell him a dozen of her finest, but only a dozen because she had to buy them that way and did not want to break up the set; presumably, this French madam, like many of her English counterparts, did a brisk side business in selling condoms in quantity.

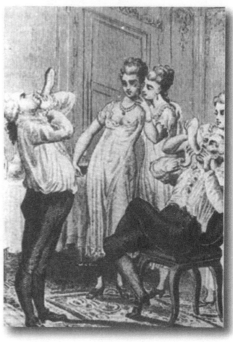

Casanova's "party trick"

Feeling he was being fleeced, Casanova made the best of the situation by requesting his *fille de joie* help him pick just which of the overpriced condoms he should wear; she "came back with the packet. I put myself in the right position, and ordered her to choose me one that fitted well. Sulkily, she began examining and measuring. . . . 'This one doesn't fit well' I told her. 'Try another.' Another, and another; and suddenly I splashed her well and truly."

Not all of Casanova's *willing* lovers appreciated his raincoats, however. One of them told him she preferred him au naturel, enjoying his "ce petit personnage" more without the "nasty, disgusting, and scandalous covering." She went on to condemn the condom as something meant only for the boring and overcautious: "Love devised these little coats, but love in alliance with caution, and that's a dull kind of alliance, fit only for gloomy politics." In spite of his obvious respect for the little item, Casanova did record that there were times when he "shut myself up in a piece of dead skin in order to prove that I am perfectly alive" and found it very unsatisfying.

By far the most entertaining account of his experiences with condoms took place while he was having an affair with a French nun. While snooping through her things, Casanova was amazed to discover a box of sheaths in her secretary. Curious to see whether she would miss them, he quietly put the box into his pocket and quickly penned a poem to put in its place. As Casanova and his lover were going to bed, she excused herself and went to her secretary to get her box. Instead of the condoms, Casanova's lover found the poem he had left in their place:

> *Children of friendship, ministers of grief,*
> *I am Love; tremble and respect the thief.*
> *And you, God's wife, shrink not from motherhood;*
> *If you conceive, He will claim fatherhood.*
> *But if you will your fruits to me deny,*
> *Speak up; I'll unman myself to comply.*

Quickly penning a reply that might leave the reader of the verse wondering why this lady had become a nun, she responded in kind:

> *When an angel fucks me I've no doubts*
> *That nature's author is my only spouse.*
> *But to keep His line above suspicion*
> *Love must return my sheaths without objection.*
> *Only as I'm subject to His holy will*
> *May my friend fuck me fearless, as he will.*

Casanova gave in, returned the box, donned a little sheath, and proceeded to unman himself. He describes how after an hour, his lover removed his sheath to gaze upon his "quintessence therein."

Casanova's lewd story adds an interesting footnote to the history of the condom. It proves that women of the eighteenth century were not just their primary manufacturers and purveyors: they also purchased them. And the fact that a nun slept with the world's most famous lover? The humble little condom cannot be blamed or credited.

◆❦❧◆

That the world is overrun with vice cannot be denied; but vice,
however predominant, has not yet gained an unlimited dominion.
Samuel Johnson in his *Rambler Essays,* 1751

Perhaps not as universally recognized as Casanova, another eighteenth-century condom chronicler is still a household name in England, famed in British history as a real ladies' man. Or at the very least a man with a penchant for having sex out-of-doors.

James Boswell was a Scottish lawyer and writer, but is best known as the biographer and dear friend of Samuel Johnson. A very prolific author himself, Dr. Johnson is second only to Shakespeare as the most quoted writer in history, and he is the father of the modern dictionary.

Perhaps most significant in the story of Boswell is that Dr. Johnson was also renowned throughout Europe as a moral philosopher, a man who sought to smite vice at every turn. In spite of his friend's influence, however, Boswell was anything but anti-vice or sexually conservative—quite the opposite; he had little regard for public, or private, morality. It is a historical irony, in fact, that the friend and biographer of a man distinguished in history for his righteous homilies and proclamations on the evils of vice was himself a sexual gladiator.

James Boswell did not begin his amorous adventures as a condom zealot. He noted in his personal journal that his first experience wearing one was not much fun. He had picked up a teenaged prostitute in St. James's Park and "For the first time did I engage in armour, which I found but a dull satisfaction."

In spite of this lack of enthusiasm for his armour, a few weeks after that first engagement he tried using it again (Boswell is also one of those who believed in getting the most for his money, wearing the same armour over and over again) and "strolled into the Park and took the first whore I met, whom without many words copulated with free from danger, being safely sheathed. She was ugly and lean and her breath smelt of spirits. When it was done, she slunk off. I had a low opinion of this gross practice and resolved to do it no more." This time his complaint was about having anonymous sex with a skinny stranger, not about using a condom.

But Boswell was a man with a very active libido, and he broke his vow to himself to "do it no more," at the same time proving his renewed dedication to the use of armour: "At the bottom of Haymarket I picked up a strong, jolly young damsel, and taking her under the arm I conducted her to Westminster Bridge, and there in armour complete did engage her upon this noble edifice. The whim of doing it there with the Thames rolling below has amused me much." He no doubt enjoyed the extra-added excitement of the possibility of being caught while *engaging* out-of-doors while all of London was in the streets that night, celebrating the birthday of King George III.

There were times when the promise of exciting sex overcame Boswell's caution. Only a few days after the "King's celebration," he recorded in his journal his next exploit: "I picked up a fresh, agreeable girl called Alice Gibbs. We went down a lane to a snug place, and I took out my armour, but she begged that I might not put it on, as the sport was much pleasanter without it, and as she was quite safe. I was so rash as to trust her, and had a very agreeable congress."

At least Boswell suffered from a fit of worry over what he might have picked up, and his remorse did the trick: he was back in his armour within a week. This time, before engaging in more alfresco sex, he took a moment to rinse it off in a canal, probably because wet gut fits better than dry, rather than because of a genuine concern over cleanliness.

. . . no voice save that of the passions can conduct you to happiness.

The Marquis de Sade

The most infamous condom user in history has to be the Marquis de Sade, who, like his slightly more conventional eighteenth-century Italian counterpart, was so well known in his own time for his sexual exploits, his name has its own special place in the English language. Unlike that of Casanova's though, the Marquis' name has a sinister air to it, as a reference to cruel or unnatural sex. Sadism. Sadist. Sadistic.

Donatien Alphonse François de Sade was from an aristocratic French family. However, in spite of his social status and his reputation as the worst of sexual libertines, he somehow managed to survive the French Revolution and the guillotine.

De Sade's entire life was devoted to his sexual exploits—and to writing about them. He used his personal experiences and those of others, real and imagined, as the basis of his writings. *Justine*, the Marquis' most famous and most controversial book, put him on the map as a novelist and a pornographer, but it is in his book *La Philosophie dans le Boudoir* (Philosophy in the Bedroom, ca. 1795) where de Sade discussed his favorite methods of birth control. One of those was the condom—or as he referred to it, "un petit sac de peau de Venise" (a little sack of the skin of Venice).

As the characters in his *Philosophie* discuss the various methods for practicing "safe sex," the gentleman patiently explains to the lady, "Others oblige their fuckers to make use of a little sack of Venetian skin, in the vulgate called a condom, which the semen fills and where it is prevented from flowing farther." The term *Venetian skin* refers to where the little sacks he favored were manufactured; Venetian makers were known to make a superior condom, and de Sade used only the best.

For his literary efforts and exploits, the Marquis de Sade was both loved and despised by his contemporaries. He is remembered today as not only a prolific writer of pornography but also for his passion for all things kinky. Eventually, though, his writings about sexual excess as well as his outrageous personal habits landed him in a French prison, accused of "crimes against nature."

In many ways the condom was in its heyday in the seventeenth and eighteenth centuries, when it was not only commonly used but was actually *de rigueur* among the elite. Condom makers tried to diversify and produce a variety of sizes and qualities. Women spoke up regarding their own preferences—on or off. And during a time in history when they had few options as far as supporting themselves, some women found producing and selling armour, sheaths, and machines an excellent way to make a living. On the flip side, it was women who suffered the gravest consequences from dirty or failed condoms and experienced the greatest discomfort from the poorly made variety.

But that is the European baudruche. What about the New World? When did the condom make its way to America?

SAUCY LOVE, PULLBACKS, AND THE GOOD DOCTOR . . . *SEX IN THE NEW WORLD*

> *. . . a fair virgin, longing to be sped*
> *and meet her lover in a nuptial bed,*
> *decked in rich ornaments to advance her state and excellence,*
> *being most fortunate when most enjoyed . . .*
>
> Thomas Morton's vision of America, 1625

In 1625, the Puritans of Plymouth Colony were shocked when the English barrister and adventurer Thomas Morton took over a plantation just down the road from the virtuous colonists. The friction was hardly surprising considering Morton's philosophy: he advocated free love for men and women and he envisioned his plantation as an oasis of sexual self-expression and exploration. He also consorted openly with the local natives, "dancing and frisking togither."

Morton's sexually charged colony-within-a-colony, aptly named Merry Mount, so offended the Puritans that in 1628 they sent Captain Miles Standish to arrest him; Morton managed to avoid Standish, but eventually they forcibly deported him back to England after Puritan leaders accused

THE NEW WORLD
From the English broadside "The Summons to New England," making fun of colonial prudery:

Loe in this Church all shall be free
To enjoy their Christian liberty;
All things made common, t' voide strife,
Each man may take another's wife,
And keep a handmaid too, if need,
To multiply, increase, and breed.

Morton and his followers of "pour[ing] themselves into all profaneness" and participating in "unclean acts."

So determined to live the unfettered lifestyle he envisioned possible in the New World, after only a short stay in England, Morton foolishly returned to his Merry Mount. He was no more welcome the second time around; upon arrival, the Puritans promptly threw him in prison, where he was so badly treated that he died soon after.

Morton's case was a precautionary tale for those from the Old World who believed they could arrive on the shores of Massachusetts and live their lives as they pleased. The Puritans were a determined group who were sure that they could keep their colony "moral" if they made all sexual acts they considered "unclean" illegal. Adultery was punishable by death and was defined as a man having sex with a married woman. And their "Buggery Laws" declared masturbation and oral sex—because they wasted the seed—crimes against God.

But no matter how hard those early settlers tried to control other people's sex lives, as the colonies expanded and matured, sexual beliefs and behaviors were as varied as the population itself, reflecting the European norms from which they derived. In

> **BUGGERY LAWS**
> The sixteenth-century English buggery laws take their name from the French slang word *bougres*, which means *heretical*.

fact, the late colonial period was a pretty sexy one. These were the folks who encouraged premarital sex with the practice of "bundling," where a couple contemplating betrothal was allowed to sleep in the same bed, with just a blanket or board between them. Religious colonials were also quite literal in discussing the duties of a wife to supply her husband with ample sex, as "the Conjugal Relation" came from "the natural Inclinations of Men, of which Himself [meaning God] is the author."

> *... a noise afrighted him and made him run away and he then carried away in haste her petticoat instead of his britches.*

Evidence of lurid behaviors, and normal sexual activity, are peppered throughout colonial and revolutionary literature. Parents wrote to sons away from home warning them against the wanton behaviors of young people, fearful of the consequences of unprotected sex. And it is the concerns themselves that document the steady loosening of moral codes in the late colonial period, especially obvious in the growing cities. Even Harvard University was the target of fear and scorn by parents worried about their children's sexual purity. A father preparing to send his son off to that hallowed institution as early as 1672 told the boy to be wary of "youthful lusts, speculative wantonness, and secret filthiness . . . do not waste . . . your precious time by love of any filthy lust." Strong language for a post-Puritan.

Interestingly, even in Governor Bradford's history of the Plymouth Colony, there are snippets from private letters and journals that indicate Americans were a fairly excitable bunch and that they practiced birth control. Like the women of earlier cultures, and of early modern Europe, married women generally took responsibility for it, and they used a variety of methods to prevent contraception or to interfere with a pregnancy. Some of these practices arrived with the Europeans, and some were learned from the Native peoples, who utilized many of the same herbal contraceptive remedies that would have been recognizable to the ancients. Men were also involved, though if Governor Bradford's accounts are anything to go by, they were more concerned about covering up their affairs with married women or with young servants than about taking responsibility when they practiced birth control.

> *Roger, rogering, love, yard, spent, clapped, manual uncleanliness,*
> *giving a flourish, taking a bout, saucy love, mowing, powerful*
> *flourish, girling of it, fuddled, flopper, enveloped, topped,*
> *fucksters . . .*
> The language of love in eighteenth-century America

Although the social constraints of the early colonial period had relaxed by the time the colonists began their struggle to be free of British control, the revolutionary period has been represented historically as a sexually constrained one. In fact, although they may have been the recipients of the Founding Fathers' high-minded ideals for nation building, many Americans lived pretty lusty lifestyles.

At *dusts* and *kick-ups* young men and women frolicked, sometimes with no chaperones. During the American Revolution, revolutionary soldiers were welcomed to join in, especially if they were of the same social status as the host and other guests. When he was able to get a girl alone, and by all accounts many young women were just as eager to *frolick* as the young men, the smart soldier, especially one who came from a nearby town or village, made attempts to prevent getting a girl pregnant. Those men who had been raised on farms or who worked as butchers would have known what their forebears had understood: the intestines of a cow, goat, or sheep could be fashioned into a useful device, when they could get hold of a length of gut. Sailors, on the other hand, had greater access to premade condoms, imported from Europe; if they had the funds, smart sailors could fill their sea chests with contraband condoms (hidden from the tax collector's view) and would have made a tidy sum selling to tavern owners and fellow sailors.

Journals and other documents from the revolutionary period, though, are not forthcoming (or specific) about condom use. There are few asides detailing the kind of activities noted in European sources, and judging by the high rate of "shotgun" marriages at the time, protection was either not as popular, or as well understood, as in Europe—or there were lots of failures. But that would change during the two or three decades following the Revolution, when the secretive condom emerged, assuming its permanent place in American history. Appropriately, it is in the new nation's first two capitals that the humble little condom began to come out of the closet.

THE DOCTOR, THE GUILLOTINE, AND THE CONDOM

In postrevolutionary Philadelphia, illicit sex was not just for the red-light districts. Casual sexual encounters and adultery were commonplace among Philadelphians of all social classes. It was probably because of its social and sexual freedoms that the nation's first capital became home to the condom's first and biggest retail market.

By the late 1700s, the City of Brotherly Love had become a retreat for a thriving French émigré community, many of the ex-patriots having escaped Robespierre and his infamous guillotine. One of the most interesting and colorful of these was Mederic Louis Elie Moreau de St. Mery, a

French lawyer born in the West Indies. When St. Mery left the islands for Paris in the 1760s, he joined the French king's gendarmerie and eventually studied law. He even claimed to have been the one to have rediscovered and restored Christopher Columbus's tomb.

When St. Mery decided in the early 1790s to tour his native Santa Domingo, he found that French politics had affected the islands and it was not safe for someone who had once worked for the king to go to the French Caribbean. Rather than cancel his plans to travel, he decided to take an extended tour of the new American nation instead.

When he arrived in America's first capital, St. Mery liked the thriving —and rowdy—city. He wrote enthusiastically about seeing President George Washington open the first Congress and was generally fascinated by the new American nation. He enjoyed the experience so much, he decided to stay.

In order to support himself, in 1794, St. Mery opened a bookshop on Front and Walnut streets where he sold "minute" books (trendy little volumes like *Poor Richard's Almanac* and brainier French works by Voltaire). However, the lawyer recognized the possibility of a much more lucrative market in the bawdy capital; along with the mostly French books he sold to his fellow émigrés, St. Mery imported fine condoms from Paris and did a thriving business selling the little items to both Frenchmen and Americans.

When he described how his business grew beyond selling just books, St. Mery recorded it this way in his diary: "I did not wish to deprive my business of a profitable item, the lack of which in hot climates would not, I think, be without danger. Consequently, when my old colleague and friend, Barrister Geanty, a refugee from Cape Francois in Baltimore, who had a wide knowledge of medical supplies, offered me a stock of certain small contrivances—ingenious things said to have been suggested by the stork— I agreed. I wish to say that I carried a complete assortment of them for four years; and while they were primarily intended for the use of French colonials, they were in great demand among Americans, in spite of the false shame so prevalent among the latter. Thus the use of this medium on the vast American continent dates from this time. People from San Domingo as well as from other colonies had frequent recourse for our stock."

Although venereal disease was epidemic in Philadelphia at the time, St.

Mery's French customers purchased their baudruches as much for birth control as for disease prevention. The demand was so great he had a hard time keeping his shelves filled. This was due in part to the fact that, though St. Mery's business was a legitimate one, his importation practices were not quite as aboveboard. He paid ships' captains to smuggle his condoms in their personal lockers, avoiding the prying eyes of customs agents and the heavy tariff the little items carried. This practice could slow down delivery. He was also convinced that only the French could make a truly fine baudruche, and he refused to set up a manufacturing business to produce his own.

> **ONLY THE FINEST**
> French-made condoms remained the most popular for centuries. It was because of their reputation for quality, but as important was their mystique, their "Frenchness." The skin variety kept their fancy appellation, goldbeaters, for centuries. One J. C. Galoupeau of New York took advantage of the age-old status and advertised his Goldbeater's Skins *as "the best article ever manufactured and imported into this market."*

His business also gave St. Mery a bird's-eye view of Philadelphian society; the Frenchman was keenly aware of the social interactions among the city's inhabitants. In spite of his excellent sales, he was very cynical about his American customers' use of the condom, as he mentioned in his diary. He felt they were hypocritical in the way they indulged; well-known, wealthy, and well-respected customers appeared very upright and conservative in public, yet they surreptitiously bought and used condoms in order to protect themselves while having adulterous affairs and making extensive use of the many prostitutes in the city. American men had never been so interested in reading before. St. Mery preferred the honest dalliances of the French upper classes.

He also noted with some disgust the general ignorance of American women regarding issues of sexuality, perhaps explaining why there is no documentation of women buying or selling condoms (unlike their European counterparts) during this period. This general ignorance about sex remained a sad fact for American women well into the twentieth century.

Unfortunately, though St. Mery was a well-respected merchant, and a member of the Philadelphia Philosophical Society where he counted among his friends and associates men like Talleyrand and French Consul

Lesseps (father of the builder of the Suez Canal), St. Mery was not a very good businessman. It was probably due then to poor business acumen rather than poor sales that in 1797 he decided to sell his business and return to France, where he was embraced by Empress Josephine; later, he was a great proponent and public advocate of the sale of Louisiana to America, assuring the French leaders that the exchange would cement American and French alliances.

St. Mery's exit from Philadelphia was a great loss to the city, but not to condom sales. By then, Philadelphians could purchase protection from barbers, madams, individual peddlers, and in taverns, as well as imported baudruches from discreet tradesmen.

THE SECOND CONDOM CAPITAL

By the 1740s and long after the American Revolution, New York's first red-light district was known as the Holy Ground, so named because the land it occupied—which was adjacent to what is today Columbia University—was owned by the Episcopal Trinity Church. Here on Holy Ground, tavern keepers and madams quietly offered condoms for sale. However, the device was most popular among middle- and upper-class men, who enjoyed the easy access and inexpensive services of a huge assortment of prostitutes—and young women who enjoyed late-night adventures with strangers—when they visited New York. Working-class men, on the other hand, rarely used protection; like Philadelphia, the class distinction is evidenced by the terrible incidence of *the clap*, *the pox*, and *the fatal disorder* suffered by working-class New Yorkers (and British soldiers during the Revolution) who partook of the Holy Ground's entertainments. Naval officers were the most likely to use condoms regularly—they had the access to imports from Europe and could afford the good quality favored by European lovers—and were more worldly than the country folk, common soldiers, and sailors who flocked to the second capital.

High-class prostitutes did ask customers to use protection, but the poor streetwalkers and brothel workers had a difficult time convincing lesser clients to use protection; they could not afford condoms themselves.

Although quietly available from private sources, they were expensive (the best sold for the equivalent of five dollars a piece on today's market). That could easily be many months' pay for a streetwalker. That and the fact that few working-class people understood the horrible possible consequences of unprotected sex, or were simply unaware of condom use, meant that protection was not taken as seriously as it was by the upper classes. However, for the "working girl," using a condom would have made a lot of sense.

Manhattan's debtor's prison was used not just to lock up unfortunates owing monies they could not repay: pimps frequently locked up their "girls" who were unlucky enough to become pregnant. And late eighteenth-century New York's hospitals and almshouses were full of prostitutes debilitated and dying from the painful symptoms of the clap and the pox.

SEVEN

malthus, skins, and dead letters

THE WEST'S CULTURE WARS

By the end of the eighteenth century, Europe and America had seen a great number of changes at home and abroad. Captain Cook had made his historic journey to the South Pole, Mozart and Haydn were writing some of history's most important pieces of music, and Coleridge, Wordsworth, and Blake were ushering in a "great age for poetry." America had broken free of British control and the French Revolution had created Europe's first constitutional government. There were also slowly emerging social movements that would eventually introduce radical social changes to Western society.

When Mary Wollstonecraft published her feminist treaty *A Vindication of the Rights of Woman*, she ushered in the long, painful struggle on the part of women to achieve social and economic parity with men. And though the new American Constitution proved to be a "great compromise" when those who argued that it should reject the institution of slavery lost their battle, the issue did not go away and abolitionism was born. But it was perhaps Malthusian theory that really launched one of the most interesting social movements of the time, one that helped shape modern Western society's approach to human sexuality.

Historians of this period often lump together all of the struggles of the late eighteenth and nineteenth centuries as the "culture wars."

Although the English and American wars were fought over different issues—England's began over the rigid social class system and the causes and solutions of poverty, whereas the American battles were fought over the institution of slavery and women's rights—both countries' struggles had one thing in common: their *skins*, *gloves*, and *letters* were front and center in the acrimonious debates over their social and political futures.

A powerful social movement began in England in 1798 with the publication of a pamphlet titled *An Essay on the Principle of Population*. Authored by ordained priest Thomas Malthus, the short tract hypothesized that as the poor and working classes increased in number, their population would eventually outstrip the available food supply. Malthus had been influenced in his beliefs by both the philosophies of his father, a gentleman of means and an avid armchair philosopher, and his father's philosophical friends, the most important being Swiss socialist philosopher Jean-Jacques Rousseau. Unlike the majority of Britons, these men believed that everyone, rich or poor, had the power of reason, no matter what social class or standing. Malthus incorporated this belief into his theory, convinced that even the poor could be convinced that they needed to curb their reproduction for the greater good.

Reaction to Malthusian theory was strong and swift: plenty of American intellectuals like Thomas Jefferson embraced the idea, but because the North American continent appeared to have endless boundaries, fear of too many poor people never got a foothold. Not so in England, however, where the theory resonated for many intellectuals, as well as middle- and upperclass Britons, who were worried about the sharp increase in the population of British poor at this time. Either way, right or wrong, the Malthusians inadvertently brought about the "birth" of the first birth control movement, and along with it came the condom.

Malthus personally thought that the solution to the looming population and ensuing food shortage crisis was for the lower classes to stop having children. He was not specific about just how to make this happen, except to have the poor use "preventative checks."

Although Malthus was not very helpful in providing specifics about just how to help the poor stop reproducing, his theory is important to this chapter in condom history. In a roundabout way, he is the father of the modern birth control movement, a movement he would not actually lead, but would foster through his mentoring of the first of the brave men who did work toward making contraception a *public matter*.

It began when Malthusian philosopher Jeremy Bentham, well known in the late eighteenth and early nineteenth centuries as an author and social activist, urged his fellow Malthusians to embrace the idea that family size limitation for the poor could only be achieved if they used birth control. A far cry from just "expecting" abstinence. Although Bentham was not in love with the condom—he condescendingly referred to it as the "dead letter"— he at least recognized the fact that if the poor were expected to use birth control, they would need to be educated about a variety of easy-to-use and easy-to-understand preventatives.

Another important voice in the movement was radical journalist and printer Richard Carlile. Best known for his antigovernment pamphlets urging Parliament to pass much-needed social and economic reforms—and his long stays in jail because of them—Carlile was also pro–women's rights. In his 1825 self-published tract, *Every Woman's Book*, or *What Is Love?* Carlile most heartily recommended that women use the *sponge* (modeled after the ancient tampon), a birth control method that had reemerged in France after at least a thousand-year hiatus, but he also talked about the skin or glove as a way in which men could help prevent pregnancy. He counseled: "These are sold in London at brothels, by waiters at taverns and by some women and girls in the neighbourhood of places of resort, such as Westminster Hall." Carlile's knowledge of the easiest places to buy condoms is notable; he also followed the movements of government officials so closely that he knew many members of Parliament were avid users of gloves and that they found it a convenience to buy their supplies on the way to running the country.

But Carlile also complained that skins were "artificial" because they could deaden sensation and were an interruption. Like the eighteenth-century physicians who preceded him, it is unclear as to whether Carlile felt this way because of personal experience or presumed it and was worried that the artificiality of condom use meant many working-class men would reject using a glove.

Either way, although men like Bentham and Carlile may sound a bit stiff and maybe even prudish, they were extremely courageous for speaking publicly to what was in many ways a sexually ignorant nation about how to limit family size; in spite of the fact that the condom had been popular in England probably since the Norman period, average Englishmen were not well educated regarding their own bodies. And the condom's modern English history was mostly associated with disease prevention. As a publicly advocated birth control device, discussing it was new and sometimes dangerous ground, which opened the Malthusians up to severe public criticism. In one of many reactions to the handbills Carlile produced and circulated about birth control, one detractor encapsulated the hypocritical attitudes about sex that were common at the time: "If the reader require anything to disgust him with the foregoing filth, let him go herd with wolves and monkeys: he is unfit for human fellowship." Everyone is a critic.

GRASSROOTS CONDOMS

The early Malthusians generally used the written word to convince the English poor of the need to practice birth control; they were well meaning, but few of their intended audience could read well or at all. There were, though, some family limitation advocates who understood the true meaning of "grassroots campaigning." Earthier and more practical in their efforts to help the poor understand birth control and its connection to alleviating poverty, early nineteenth-century condom adherents also used written tracts to spread the word, but their pamphlets were not lofty lectures on the need to limit population to spare the human race; they instructed the reader on how to make condoms.

The "receipts" were written in the simplest terms, with directions about purchasing animal intestines from a butcher (with assurances that the butcher need not know the purpose of the purchase!) and then how to fashion condoms out of the material. The recipes were distributed in the poorer sections of London and the larger northern cities. Whether they had much impact is another issue, but it would have been amusing to see upper-class matrons, determined to help mankind, handing out illustrated instructions on how to make gloves.

RECIPES FOR MAKING CONDOMS

1824 *Ordinary condoms are made from sheeps intestinal caeca soaked in water for some hours, turned inside out, macerated again in weak alkaline changed every 12 hours, scraped carefully to remove the mucous membrane, leaving the peritoneal and muscular coats; exposed to the vapour of burning brimstone, washed with soap and water; blown up, dried, cut to length of 7–8 inches, bordered at the open end with a riband.*

Baudruches fines; soaked in weak ley, turned inside out, dressed as before. Soaked in ley again, brimstoned, drawn smooth upon oiled moulds of a proper size, with the external coast of the gut next to the mould.

Baudruches superfines; washed in 2 soapy waters after soaking in them for 24 hours and very carefully dressed with the knife. Soaked in hard water for 3 days, the water being often changed; dried with a clean cloth, scented with essences, and being stretched on a glass mould, rubbed with a glass to polish them. Condoms should be soaked in water before use to make them supple.

1844 *Take the caecum of the sheep; soak it first in water, turn it on both sides, then repeat the operation in a weak ley of soda, which must be changed every four or five hours, for five or six successive times; then remove the mucous membrane with the nail; sulphur, wash in clean water, and then in soap and water; rinse, inflate and dry. Next cut it to the required length, and attach a piece of ribbon to the open end. Used to prevent infection or pregnancy. The different qualities consist in extra pains being taken in the above process, and in polishing, scenting, etc.*

GOD GAVE US BEARDS

By the 1840s, British newspapers had gotten into the birth control act, boldly carrying ads for condoms and other birth control devices and methods. Probably the most colorful and entertaining of all the advertisements was written by someone who identified himself only as "a Married Man with Six Children!"

GREY'S PHARMACOPOEIA

The 1828 edition of Gray's Supplement to the Pharmacopoeia gives a more detailed description of how sheep's intestine (caeca or cecum) was used to produce condoms. The machines were made of an "extraordinary fine thin Substance," usually the dried gut of a sheep. Also commonly used were the intestines of lambs, calves, and goats. The subheading for this illuminating description was "Condoms, Armour, baudruches, redingotes Anglaises."

In *On the Use of Night-Caps*, which was written to appear to be a legitimate editorial, Married Man takes to task the small group of birth control advocates who preached *coitus interuptus* as the best method: "How a gentleman . . . could make a practice, in the very moment of unutterable ecstasy, of withdrawing from the arena, is more than I can conceive." He went on to suggest that the best course of action was to place "over the gentleman's gentleman a very fine nightcap, doing little to dull the sensation."

The reader was notified that this creative salesman's *night-caps* were a "simple French invention . . . universally known in France." And he suggested that though a *wife* was likely to laugh when she first saw the "*French letter*, why not let her help him try it on?" As one who believed in making the condom a part of foreplay, Casanova would have been proud of Married Man: "Let it be tried *on*, and the experiment would be found not complete without its being tried *in*. At one of the numerous contacts most married people enjoy, this experiment would be interesting from its novelty." The writer then assured his reader that this does not have to be done until the last minute and will not disturb the process, since it takes only a few seconds. Pity the Malthusians did not know this.

In his thorough sales pitch, Married Man also tried to reassure the moralists who might condemn condoms on ethical grounds. He mentions the fact that the *night-cap* cannot be used for "seduction" because no "virgin could be opened by a gentleman's member, with the cap on, without its bursting." It is hard enough to imagine a modern newspaper like the *Washington Post* accepting this kind of explicit advertisement today, but in 1840s England?

In his final attempt to cover any and all objections his audience might have had to using a condom—specifically those concerns about the moral rights and wrongs of birth control—our writer makes this marvelous analogy: "God gave us beards, but man invented razors."

AMERICA'S CULTURE WARS

Although America did not suffer the crowding and therefore the population debates of Europe, beginning in the early part of the nineteenth century it did have its own battles over social issues: America's culture wars were fought over gender roles, racism and slavery, socioeconomic issues . . . and sex.

One of the loudest voices in the battle over the rights and wrongs of birth control and human sexuality was Scottish-born Robert Dale Owen. Owen moved to England as a child, and at the age of twenty-four, he emigrated to America with his father, Robert Owen Sr., who is famous in American history as the founder of New Harmony, a utopian community in Illinois. The younger Owen inherited his activist spirit from his father, who had hoped that by creating a self-sustaining community dedicated to cooperation and rational education, he could fix what was wrong with the world. Among his other claims to fame, Owen was also one of the founders of the Smithsonian Institute in Washington, DC, served as a member of the House of Representatives, and was a tireless advocate who pushed the federal government to fund public education. But he was also a strong advocate for free and legal birth control.

Owen returned to England regularly in the first few decades of the nineteenth century and on one of his trips he read Carlile's tract on birth control, bringing at least one copy back to the United States. It was the influence of the English activists, especially Carlile, that led to Owen becoming America's first birth control advocate.

As far as the actual methods he favored, Owen believed that coitus interuptus was the safest, but he also talked about the condom or "a covering made of very fine, smooth, and delicately prepared skin." His greatest concern was that condoms were not a very clean method and complained that they were inconvenient and expensive, "a baudruche being fit for use once only, and costing about a dollar." Owen obviously had not been exposed to the linen or silk condoms still available in his native country, where men still washed and reused their gloves.

His methods were assailed by advocates of women's rights as impractical, in fact, down right chauvinistic, giving men all the power when it came to deciding when, if, and what to use. But as with his English counterparts, Owen is best viewed through the lens of his own times: in his final summation of the condom and of birth control in general—and in spite of his prejudices—he felt that the glove was perfectly moral and "innocent." And his final answer to women advocates whose objection to the condom was that it put all the control in the hands of men? A woman's ultimate and "only effectual defence" was to "refuse connexion with any man void of honour." Simple enough!

Joining the ranks of birth control advocates were a handful of medical professionals who spoke publicly about birth control methods, including men like Massachusetts physician Charles Knowlton. Knowlton broke scientific ground when he called contraception a moral right and he worked hard to educate the general public as to "what worked." But Knowlton was against the condom because he felt it was an unhealthy and expensive contraceptive method, "on account of cleanliness and expense . . . and by no means calculated to some into general use"; yet like others, he continued to identify it with disease prevention, or "syphilitic affections."

Although Knowlton is another good example of the activists who believed information about contraception should be readily available to the masses, historically his work is more important as an example of the somewhat schizophrenic public and legal approach to human sexuality that was prevalent in early nineteenth-century America.

Many average Americans were desperate for birth control advice, and the open marketplace had been trying to address the need for many decades. Especially in large cities, Americans were becoming more open about sex in general, but what the public wanted was not always reflected in the legal realm, especially when it came to condoms. Charles Knowlton was arrested for indecency and sentenced to three months hard labor just for writing about them. This was not his first arrest; the first time Knowlton was sent to prison was for "illegal dissection." He had stolen a corpse from a cemetery so that he could study and write about the human body. Sadly, Knowlton's arrest early in the century foreshadowed what would happen more than four decades later under the guise of protecting public morality.

SEX IN THE LYCEUM

In spite of the sporadic legal prosecutions of birth control advisers (not those who actually made and sold condoms), beginning in the 1820s and continuing until the 1870s, writers and lecturers including Ralph Waldo

Emerson traveled all over the growing country, speaking to audiences about physiology and all manner of sexual matters.

Important and highly charged issues of the time, as well as much more benign subjects, found an eager audience in the lyceum and along the local lecture circuits. Especially during the winter months, urban Americans were desperate for diversion and would happily pay a few cents to hear professionals discuss their fields, as well as to listen to social activists trying to find support for their causes. In this atmosphere, the condom found a cozy niche in lectures about human sexuality.

Among the speakers of the day were self-styled "sex experts" who took full advantage of public curiosity and a *need to know*. The experts were not doctors or scientists, but a motley group of supporters of the women's rights and abolitionist movements as well as savvy businesspeople. But no matter the motives of the experts, they took full advantage of what St. Mery, America's first *condom professional*, had noted in his keen observations of Americans and sexuality: they were, especially women, ignorant of even the fundamentals regarding their own bodies.

The popularity of this first wave of public discourses on sex, the human body, and contraception was fueled by the simple desire to understand how individuals could take control of their own reproductive systems. Although many of the ladies expressed a reluctance about being seen entering a hall full of others who were sexually curious, desperate, or simply hoping to hear or see something a bit risqué, the sex lectures were some of the best attended public entertainments of the antebellum era, and continued to be popular until the early 1870s.

A number of the lecturers included in their talks specifics on how to prevent pregnancy by using sponges, douches, and condoms. After each lecture, these experts would remain on hand to peddle not only booklets they had written on the subject but also the devices about which they had lectured. Especially popular with the sex lecturers, probably because of the size and ease of transport, were condoms.

Other lecturers were actually professionals in the condom industry, advertising not only their services as traveling sex educators but also their contraceptive wares. Newspapers and broadsides publicized both, and many of the pros had thriving mail-order condom businesses. One of these used a rather unique marketing technique in his mail-order business. First he charged an unbelievable five dollars for a box of three sheaths, and he required that each order include a written explanation of why the customer needed them. Perhaps this was a marketing tool to help him in his advertising, or maybe he just found the descriptions enjoyable reading.

Possibly the most surprising of the lecture-circuit sex experts were the women, especially early feminist and Quaker Mary Gove. Gove chose the unusual itinerant lifestyle after she had found out how difficult it was to earn her own living when she had escaped an unhappy marriage. She fell back on her knowledge of anatomy and physiology—which she had studied extensively—and became genuinely interested in teaching people, especially other women, about their own reproductive systems. She had picked up sufficient knowledge in what was then state-of-the-art scientific theory to speak fairly accurately and at length about many issues pertaining to sex and the human body.

With great dignity, Gove would calmly climb the stairs to the dais, in front of often-huge audiences. In her plain Quaker dress, she reached out to other women with her straightforward speech. Gove often drew shocked gasps when she used, rather than a primitive mannequin, her own (fully clothed) body to demonstrate her points about the female anatomy. Although she had her critics, even the male-dominated medical community commended her efforts to educate women about their own sexuality, including birth control. She became so well known in fact that a medical journal wrote about her work, praising it as "nothing objectionable or indelicate for one woman to tell another those important facts . . . in a country where ladies have been too negligent of the laws of health, and sometimes apparently proud of being profoundly ignorant of the mechanism of themselves."

Among other earthy advice, Gove told men and women about the rhythm method and the use of "delicate coverings of the whole penis." At some point, she began to carry a supply of the delicate coverings with her, making a little bit extra on the side.

Surprisingly, Elizabeth Blackwell, America's most famous woman doctor, was very critical of Gove and the others who carried the contraceptive message to average Americans, accusing them of spreading doctrines of "abortion and prostitution under spiritual and scientific guise." This incorrect condemnation of their profession and purpose, however, did little to slow down the sex experts.

MR. GOODYEAR'S RUBBER AND THE GOD OF FIRE

By the late eighteenth century, Europeans who had traveled throughout South America had seen native peoples playing with soft, pliable balls made from the coagulated sap of a variety of native trees. The English discovered that bits of the soft substance, alternatively called *gutta percha* and *India rubber*, but mostly referred to just as *rubber*, could erase pencil marks. Beyond that, although both American and British manufacturers tried to turn the substance into practical items like waterproof clothing, rubber just did not stand up to changes in temperature. It took a determined and eccentric young American inventor to revolutionize its production.

Charles Goodyear was obsessed with rubber and spent years, and all his money, trying to find a way to stabilize it. Although a flexible, waterproof material, rubber was unstable, going brittle in cold weather and turning into a smelly, gelatinous mess in the heat. When manufacturers, including Goodyear, used it to produce umbrellas, boots, and other consumer goods, they found that rubber simply could not be used to make long-wearing products. Customers returned the items, disgusted with the shoddy goods that had been passed off as waterproof. But after years of experiments that actually bankrupted his family, Charles Goodyear finally realized his dream; he discovered, quite by accident, how to stabilize the sap he was so obsessed with and received his first patent for "vulcanizing" (from Vulcan, the Roman god of fire) rubber in 1837.

Vulcanization is the process of treating crude rubber with sulfur and intense heat, which turns it

NOM DE LA CONDOM

French explorer and physicist Charles de la Condamine is credited with discovering rubber while on a scientific exploration of the Amazon in the 1730s. He noted the natives tapping rubber trees—from the many varieties of Hevea—making leakproof containers, rubber balls for sports, and a type of glue. Condamine brought rubber back to France and it made its way to England, where Sir Joseph Priestley, the discoverer of oxygen, noted that it was also useful for erasing pencil marks from paper. However, it was an American from Philadelphia, Hyman Lipman, who was the first to add an eraser to a pencil. In British English an eraser is still a rubber, somewhat confusing as so is the condom. As far as the name "Condamine"? An interesting coincidence.

POVERTY AND COFFEE-TABLE BOOKS

Dedication did not make Charles Goodyear a rich man: he died in poverty, having spent every penny he had in trying to perfect his creation. Interestingly, in the coffee-table book of the History of the Goodyear Company, there is nothing mentioned about his sacrifice, or the company's huge role in producing and popularizing "the rubber." He would probably have found it a wonderful twist of fate that the company that still bears his name is now owned by another nineteenth-century upstart: Dunlop, which owns Ansell, is one of the world's largest manufacturers of twenty-first-century rubbers.

into a strong elastic material, impervious to heat or cold. The newly developed method created a stronger, more elastic, and far more durable rubber material, with the potential of making all kinds of products—including condoms.

It took about twenty years for the rubber industry to establish itself as a major player in the growing world of manufacturing, but by the late 1850s, firms like Goodyear (named after but not owned by Charles Goodyear), B. F. Goodrich, and Hancock were household names; and long before the production of tires, they were all making diaphragms, dildos (really!), and condoms. Although it stretches the imagination to envision proper ladies, dressed as if straight out of *Godey's*, going to the local hardware or general store, deciding on which dildo to purchase, or which brand of rubber was best, it happened; others preferred to order through the mail. Even the name of the basic material became an international euphemism for the condom—by the end of the nineteenth century, the English, Americans, Australians, South Americans, and many others referred to using a rubber, the nickname Goodyear himself was supposed to have given the vulcanized device.

CHARLES GOODYEAR'S DESCRIPTION OF THE FIRST RUBBER RUBBERS

When filled with water, the condom has the shape, either of an egg from which a small section has been cut, or of the glans penis. At the open end the membrane is thicker and forms a ring which holds it on. When the condom is in use this ring fits so tightly around the glans that the condom cannot slip off during intercourse, since the ring cannot pass the corona glandis.

The first rubbers resembled an industrial version of Fallopio's linen sheath; they were meant to fit over only the top of the penis, which meant greater sensitivity. The early caps had to be measured to the individual user and custom made, meaning a trip to the doctor for "fitting," which limited their popularity. They also tended to fall off at crucial moments. In answer to these concerns, it did not take long for the manufacturers to design a full-length rubber; these were available in pharmacies, one-size-fits-all. (British manufacturers were the first to offer three different sizes.)

But how comfortable were rubbers? The boasts of some manufacturers that their brands would "last for a lifetime"—as long as the wearer washed and dried his cap after each use—is evidence of not just durability but of how tough and uncomfortable early rubbers must have been. Even by the twentieth century, one rubber was often touted as being all a man would ever have to purchase; washing and drying were still the standard directive, with the added advice that slathering the condom with lots of Vaseline before putting it away would add years to its life. And although Casanova and Boswell sometimes complained about being "shut up in a dead skin," they would have hated rubbers; their armour made of animal bladder was far more "delicate." At least rubbers came in their own little leather boxes.

Though rubber sales steadily rose as the century wore on, Vulcan's condom, cap or rubber, was never as popular as the skin variety. Skins and gloves continued to be manufactured at home and by individual entrepreneurs, and were favored for their cost effectiveness and their greater sensitivity. There were also very high-quality varieties available: a package of good-quality fish-bladder "membraneous envelopes" was available for as little as five dollars a dozen—still out of the average man's price range. The very best continued to be imported from Paris and Venice, most commonly smuggled in by sea captains and small importers who did not want to pay the customs agents the high taxes condoms fetched.

GUTS VERSUS RUBBERS

In the nineteenth century, in spite of the invention of rubber condoms, which were commonly available by the 1850s, most manufacturers made their products from animal intestines imported from the large and well-established European meat processors. In fact, even after the American Civil War, US manufacturers bought ever-increasing amounts of intestines from European sausage provisioners yearly. By the 1870s, they were spending over forty-five thousand dollars a year on lamb, sheep, and cow intestines.

The reason for the need to import so much was that prior to the 1870s, there were no refrigerated railcars and meat products were locally prepared; the sausage-making—and intestine-preparing—trade was very slow to develop. A ready supply of bulk condom-making materials was not always available; plus, the Europeans had had professional baudruche manufacturers for centuries, and there were still many in the meat trade who prepared quantities of high-grade material for those not intending to make sausage.

This does not mean, however, that local American butchers did not play a role. Because the condom never achieved—nor will it—a comfortable place in people's daily speech, customers who wanted to produce their own sheaths would ask the butcher for cow or sheep intestines, carefully explaining they were making home-made sausages. As in England, by the 1840s, recipes for making condoms were being widely circulated in the big cities, begun by an anonymous birth control advocate in Philadelphia, then spreading to small towns, and throughout farming communities along the eastern seaboard.

TAXES AND TARRIFFS

Prefabricated condoms coming from Paris had carried a high tariff since the 1790s, but not so the refined European gut from which they were made. That material remained a favorite of American manufacturers through to the end of the nineteenth century, affordable because of the low tariffs that had been demanded by certain American producers who used their political clout to keep certain import taxes low; skins and hides were one of the protected imports, and fortunately the guts fell loosely under that category.

DON'T FORGET YOUR FRENCH LETTERS!

In 1840s America, professionally made condoms were available in a variety of styles, and the desired quality dictated the manufacturing process. A throwback from early condom making, the most expensive on the market were "goldbeaters," inferring a very fine texture and fit. The untreated intestinal material was put through a lengthy series of chemical processes, expertly molded, and smothered with oil. The cheapest (and those made at home) were slices of dried intestine, glued or sewn together, and tied at the top with ribbon or a piece of scrap fabric.

The popularity of skins and rubbers—commercially made, imported, or homemade—continued to grow during and immediately following the Civil War. Here again there is a historical switch that takes place regarding why men wore condoms: from the late eighteenth century until the war, the condom had been talked about, condemned, and lauded as a birth control device. But during and after the 1860s, partly because of the displacement of so many men from their homes and communities, partly because of the impoverishment of so many young women left without the support of their men and with no promise of real jobs or decent employment—and because of the dramatic population shift to the cities—there was a huge increase in prostitution during this period. The clap and the pox reemerged as public

SURE CURE.—DR. POWERS, SUCCESSFULLY consulted with Dr. WARD, No. 12 Laight-st. He gives advice free and guarantees an immediate cure or no pay. Glorious triumph of medicine. Dr. POWERS' sure specific remedies for syphilitic, mercurial and all other delicate diseases; for certainty unapproached, and for the entire eradication of disease nothing besides can positively be relied upon; try them and be convinced. Dr. POWERS' Essence of Life restores the vigor of youth in four weeks. This marvelous agent restores manhood to the most shattered constitutions. Office No. 12 Laight-st. Dr. POWERS' French Preventive, the greatest invention of the age. Those who have used them are never without them. Price, $5 per dozen; mailed free on receipt of the price. Address Dr. POWERS, No. 12 Laight-st.

Dr. Powers' "Sure Cure" condoms

health threats, and some men once again became concerned with protecting themselves and used rubbers, gloves, and French letters to avoid infection.

Even the *New York Times* got into the condom act; it was the first major American newspaper to print an advertisement for the little items. Until the 1980s, no single publication of a condom ad had the exposure the 1861 "Dr. Powers' French Preventatives" did. In fact, condoms were so readily available by then, that the cost had dropped to a mere dime apiece ($1.60 today, adjusting for inflation).

CULTURAL CONFLICT AND THE CONDOM

Partly because of the increasing access to contraceptives, as the nineteenth century progressed, the condom's role in the struggle over morality versus practicality in human sexuality was well established. On the one hand, men had been using the device to prevent disease and pregnancy for thousands of years. On the other, the nineteenth century experienced extreme social and religious movements, backlashes against changing social and economic dynamics, and frustrations over the old social and economic order, specifically women's rights and slavery. Industry, profit, and urbanization were overtaking the rural, traditional way of life. As this happened, procreation became for some a symbol of the old traditions; for those fearful of the rapid changes taking place, birth control increasingly became a symbol of immoral, loose behaviors and represented what was wrong with modern American society.

For the next 150 years, the life of the condom reflected the ups and downs of the American psyche. Some observers will read these ups and downs as reflective of a certain, or continued, cultural hypocrisy. In spite of the creeping conservatism taking hold by the mid-nineteenth century, though, rubber condoms went mainstream, making millions of dollars for manufacturers. And skins continued to be produced in greater and greater numbers. They were here to stay, but not without a fight.

EIGHT

a one-man fight against the condom

THE AMERICAN CIVIL WAR
AND COMSTOCKERY

The American Civil War certainly helped shape the last quarter of the nineteenth century, leaving the Southern portion of the nation so impoverished that it took more than a hundred years to recover. But for the rest of the nation, this era was one of the most dynamic in US history, issuing in changes, great and small, that would alter the course of American and even world history.

In 1861, Yale University awarded the first-ever American doctorate of philosophy, and that same year, the telegraph rendered the beloved Pony Express obsolete. Northerners could spend their new federally backed paper money with peace of mind, and people living in the big cities enjoyed having their mail delivered to their homes. At the close of the war, Samuel Clemens, writing as Mark Twain, was well established in the hearts and minds of American readers; Horatio Alger was doing a brisk business with his rags-to-riches novels; and Louisa May Alcott wrote what would become one of the most recognized classic novels in American history: *Little Women*. More dramatically, the United States began a crash course in international imperialism by taking pieces of the South Pacific and Asia under its wing, actions that reverberated throughout the world.

As early as 1865, however, some Americans were disturbed by the massive changes the Civil War and continuing industrialization had wrought upon the country, not just physically and politically, but socially as well. The mass migration to the cities continued at breakneck speed throughout the rest of the century and fueled an already established fear—the fear that the moral character of the nation was at risk. Cities, after all, bred moral as well as fiscal corruption. This new mood led to some astounding events and had a huge impact on the condom.

THE AMERICAN CIVIL WAR

By 1862, Washington, DC, had 450 bordellos and more than 7,500 prostitutes vying for trade. One area in particular was the favorite haunt of the Union soldiers posted to the capital city. Whether it was because their leader General Hooker—"Fighting Joe" was well known for his love of partying— and his men spent so much time there or because he actually tried to cordon it off to keep the prostitutes in one police-able place is not known, but Lafayette Square was fondly dubbed "Hooker Row." Since the term "hooker" is still a common American slang word, and was coined by the prostitutes themselves, it seems likely the latter is true. And judging by the fact that over 170,000 cases of venereal disease were treated by Union physicians during the war, many of the men who spent time with Hooker's hookers did not avail themselves of those catalog condoms.

Like militaries before them, along with food, water, munitions, and the other necessities in their rucksacks, Union and Confederate soldiers also carried their French letters, sheaths, and gloves. They were also the major market share for the booming new trade in pornographic

THE BLUE AND THE GRAY

Southerners were almost as likely to use condoms as Northerners. In cities like Richmond— where Trojans are still made—it was simple enough to buy a supply, and New Orleans was one of the easiest places to find Parisian-made baudruches. Convenience did not help a famous soldier, however. While on leave in 1861, Confederate General William Dorsey Pender's condom failed and his wife wrote to inform him that "unfortunately" she was "expecting." Pender wrote back, piously claiming that it was all "God's will" and everything would be "alright." In the same letter he included pills from his own surgeon who assured the general—who assured his wife—that the drugs would "relieve her."

photographs and novels, ordered through New York–based catalogs, the same source many military men used to buy their condoms.

But this easy sexual trade was not necessarily reflective of the attitudes of all Americans at the close of the war. In a backlash against the growing porn trade, specifically the mail-order kind, Congress was under some public pressure to pass an obscenity law intended to prevent smutty materials from being sent through the mail. At the same time, federal bureaucrats were trying to actually define just what the word *obscenity* meant. Into this odd mix of sex in the marketplace and concerns over the moral fiber of the nation stumbled an unlikely crusader.

> **Social vice and national decay were to each other as parent and child . . .**

WHO WAS ANTHONY COMSTOCK?

Anthony Comstock, an unemployed, former Union soldier, looms large in the remarkable history of the condom. A self-styled moralist who could not seem to find his professional niche in life, Comstock ended up at the center of a controversial law that plagued condom manufacturers well into the twentieth century, as well as anyone who sought, talked, wrote about, or provided information relating to human sexuality. He also played a central role in making contraception and venereal disease prevention illegal in the United States.

But where did a nobody like Comstock, a man with little education or profession, manage to secure such power? Some might argue it was his tenacity and absolute commitment to what he felt was right—a morally driven "fire in his belly"—that led him to power. But perhaps it was simply serendipity. Had some of New York's most powerful businessmen not been behind him, Comstock would probably, at best, be a historical footnote alongside the other fanatics and do-gooders who at different intervals in history have tried to rid society of its sins. It is certainly true that the history of the humble condom would have been a very different one without him.

Comstock was a devout Congregationalist from Connecticut, who during his short stint as a Union soldier offended his fellow soldiers when he slowly and deliberately poured his daily ration of whiskey onto the ground, illustrating his disgust with all things sinful. The soldiers were less concerned with his theatrics than with his wastefulness, but early on Comstock had a flair for the melodramatic. A flair he employed in his crusade against sin.

After the war, a restless and unemployed Comstock moved to New York City, shifting from one low-level job to the next. But it was being forced to live in a poor boardinghouse near the Tenderloin district, a haven for prostitutes and pimps, that pushed Comstock from being just a discontented prude to a public activist; he was so shocked at what he saw on the streets, he became obsessed with "cleaning it up."

There is no doubt that the Tenderloin was one of the most notorious neighborhoods in New York, and by the 1840s, New York itself had been dubbed the "Gomorrah of the New World." In and around the streets, Comstock walked where theaters had nude models acting out famous paintings, prostitutes offered something for everyone, and street vendors peddled smutty photographs, racy newspapers, pornographic books—and plenty of condoms.

Someone as obsessed with public morality as Comstock would have been stunned by this open "sex market." Shocked or not, though, Comstock was up for the challenge, and not long after taking up residence in a lowly boardinghouse, he began his career as a moral crusader, trolling the streets and alleyways in search of sin. When he found sin but could not get the New York City Police Department interested in arresting prostitutes and condom traders, he decided it was his civic duty to do the job for them. He hit the streets and began making citizen's arrests.

Playing the part of a kooky eccentric and brandishing his umbrella in the air while chasing after surprised prostitutes was a far cry though from becoming the man responsible for sweeping social legislation. But it was this unorthodox behavior that brought him to the attention of a wealthy New York businessman and launched his moral crusade.

Hearing about Comstock's one-man police force, Morris Jessup, also a Congregationalist originally from Connecticut, contacted Comstock. What Jessup saw when they met was a tall, imposing figure with mutton-chop sideburns and an unflinching gaze; he liked what he saw, and after that the future success of *Comstockery* was pretty much assured.

Jessup got together a group of his fellow wealthy industrialists who were all in agreement that America was fast becoming a sinful fleshpot, and they formed an offshoot of the YMCA: the NYCSV, or the New York Committee for the Suppression of Vice. Similar agencies were popping up all over the country, backed by purity crusaders who were often people of wealth: wealth derived from the urban expansion, social changes, and the working classes the crusaders so feared. People like Samuel Colgate, the great soap giant, and J. Pierpont Morgan, copper magnate and financier, were all behind the purity movement. And behind Anthony Comstock. After its creation, it did not take much effort for Comstock to get himself hired as the NYCSV's secretary, accompanied by a handsome salary that must have been very appealing to a man who had no profession or skills. Comstock loved his new job.

THE COMSTOCK ACT

Be it enacted . . . That whoever, within the District of Columbia or any of the Territories of the United States . . . shall sell . . . or shall offer to sell, or to lend, or to give away, or in any manner to exhibit, or shall otherwise publish or offer to publish in any manner, or shall have in his possession, for any such purpose or purposes, an obscene book, pamphlet, paper, writing, advertisement, circular, print, picture, drawing or other representation, figure, or image on or of paper of other material, or any cast instrument, or other article of an immoral nature, or any drug or medicine, or any article whatever, for the prevention of conception, or for causing unlawful abortion, or shall advertise the same for sale, or shall write or print, or cause to be written or printed, any card, circular, book, pamphlet, advertisement, or notice of any kind, stating when, where, how, or of whom, or by what means, any of the articles in this section . . . can be purchased or obtained, or shall manufacture, draw, or print, or in any wise make any of such articles, shall be deemed guilty of a misdemeanor, and on conviction thereof in any court of the United States . . . he shall be imprisoned at hard labor in the penitentiary for not less than six months nor more than five years for each offense, or fined not less than one hundred dollars nor more than two thousand dollars, with costs of court.

With the help of this handful of wealthy ultraconservative New York businessmen determined to make America *moral again*, Comstock also managed to make the most out of their political strengths. Morgan and others influenced some powerful Washington legislators in the Forty-second Congress to pass legislation that would, little did they know, deeply influence the nature of American sexuality.

The *Comstock Act*, as this legislation came to be called, was actually one small section of a massive postal bill, initially meant to target mail-order pornographers, something the earlier law was intended to achieve and had not, but it ended up to be a much more sweeping bill outlawing any "article of an immoral nature, or any drug or medicine, or any article whatever for the prevention of conception."

In spite of the power Comstock and his backers yielded, it was again good luck that assured the passing of the Comstock Act. The Forty-second Congress was one of the most corrupt in American history, and on the eve of President Grant's inauguration in March 1873, this Congress found itself under pressure to actually *legislate*. In the wee hours of the morning of March 3, they passed hundreds of bills, most unread by the congressmen voting for them. The postal bill was just one of the many that were pushed through that morning.

After its passage, Comstock used his powerful friends to get himself appointed as special agent of the US Post Office, the agency empowered through the new legislation to prevent obscene materials from being mailed. Under the guise of the Comstock Act—Section 211 of the Federal Criminal Code—he stretched his power to personally harass anyone who had anything to do with teaching about contraception, selling or producing birth control devices, or even discussing sex. From 1873 until just before his death in 1915, Comstock used the act to arrest 3,873 people. More than 2,900 were convicted.

✦✦✦

Comstock was passionate about his job, wielding his authority against anyone he knew was immoral or indecent, but he had an especially active dislike of condoms, condom manufacturers, and booklets about birth control. He was so *anticondom* that raiding the homes and factories of manufacturers, specifically those based in New York City, became an obsession. He was not shy about throwing the book at anyone who had an interest in them. The penalty for being caught talking about, writing about, selling, or producing condoms was prison and up to a six-hundred-dollar fine.

It is difficult to envision this man who was so dismayed by vice employing the tactics he did in order to achieve his ends: besides his standard raids and harassment,

SHAW ON COMSTOCKERY

Comstockery is the world's standing joke at the expense of the United States. Europe likes to hear of such things. It confirms the deep-seated conviction of the Old World that America is a provincial place, a second-rate country-town civilization after all.

George Bernard Shaw

PRACTICE WHAT YOU PREACH

Godfrey Lowell Cabot, a member of the powerful Brahman Cabot family and Anthony Comstock's counterpart in Boston, was almost as passionate as Comstock in his personal battle against smut. But in private he enjoyed nothing more than making extreme demands upon his wife—leading her to complain that one of her greatest unfulfilled ambitions was to have her own bedroom or at least a separate bed "where she could escape from Godfrey's sexual demands." He also wrote pornographic letters, in German, to her.

Comstock also did things like pay prostitutes to walk past him in the nude so that he could arrest them. Perhaps Comstock had a few sexual proclivities of his own, since walking around naked had nothing to do with the mail or with contraception, but his actions illustrate the ways in which Comstock abused his powers by using entrapment, a trick he employed regularly.

Whatever it was that was going on in his psyche, the Congregationalist who once told a magazine reporter that he felt "You must hunt these men [and apparently women] as you hunt rats, without mercy," helped fashion not a morally refreshed nation, but extended a long era of increased sexual hypocrisy, where the laws and the formal mores of American society did not mesh with private practice.

But Comstock never relented in his obsessive moral quest, even in his seniority. Not long before his death, he was asked by a reporter from *Harper's Weekly* why he had included condoms and other contraceptives in

ORIGINS OF PURITY

The first purity reform movement in America took place in seventeenth-century Boston. Cotton Mather founded the Society for the Suppression of Disorder in an attempt to get rid of Boston's brothels, but perhaps because he tried to combine that with also eliminating Sunday drinking and gambling, he was asking far too much of Bostonians. Even the sons and daughters of Puritans had to have their fun.

a pornography law—after all, his interviewer pointed out, the European scientific community had long ago agreed that they were important to public health. Comstock answered stubbornly: "If you open the door to anything, the filth will all pour in and the degradation of youth will follow."

DID COMSTOCK KILL THE RUBBER?

Although many arrests were made under Section 211, most (over 50 percent) were in New York City and the immediate area. As it turned out, there were far too few postal agents to be able to police the entire country—which helps explain the underground sex and birth control trade that actually flourished under Comstock's watchful eye.

Although there was risk involved, small manufacturers continued to produce and sell condoms, as well as other contraceptives. They simply changed their tactics. In discrete ads, the condom and the French letter became the *cap, sheath, capote, pouch, male shield,* or simply the *rubber good.* The best continued to be imported from Europe, smuggled in just as they had been a hundred years before.

At the turn of the twentieth century, one enterprising inventor from Texas even received a patent on his version of a "pouch" and was honest on his patent application when he described his invention as something to "catch and retain all discharges coming" from the "male member."

Amazingly, many condom sellers remained in business and even flourished. In spite of the legal consequences if they were caught, small entrepreneurs went where the larger rubber manufacturers could not go. Creating tiny condom factories, usually in their own homes, these businesses continued to provide condoms to Americans desperate for birth control, and to a lesser extent, disease prevention. They were careful to keep their stocks well

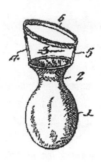

Fig. 1.

*Patent office drawing of
Ezell's "male pouch"*

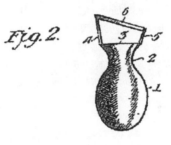

Fig. 2.

U.D. Ezell.

Geo. Ackman Jr.

Victor J. Evans

hidden, and though it is impossible to figure out just who sold how many to whom, even European travelers traversing the country during the last quarter of the nineteenth century commented in letters home about the fact that every little village seemed to have contraceptive "wares" available.

Also interesting is the fact that some of Comstock's fellow NYCSV members, and early backers, actually manufactured contraceptives. Samuel Colgate's soap company sold Vaseline, and right after the passage of the Comstock Act, Colgate began a huge advertising campaign touting his petroleum jelly (mixed with a little salicylic acid) as a *safe* contraceptive method—safe yes, contraceptive no. Goodyear, Goodrich, and Sears and Roebuck also advertised their contraceptive products in their own and others' catalogs. None of the major producers, however, were ever prose-

DESCRIPTION OF THE SMALL CONDOM FACTORY

Many smaller manufacturers continued to use animal intestines as their fabric of choice; once "cooked" it was easy to work with and the preparation of the material could be done in any home kitchen, albeit with serious dangers to their health. Producers who made rubbers were the most likely to set up shop in little rented rooms, basements, or storage areas, areas they could devote solely to their operations. There they would have a table or two, a place to hang up the rolls of rubber sheeting, and enough elbow room for a small group of employees to work. Typically, the workers—more often than not women—cut out the rubber into different sizes, fashioned each strip around penis-shaped molds made out of glass, porcelain, or hard clay, and then dipped them into a chemical solution to cure the rubber. Supplies were readily available and inexpensive, workers were a dime a dozen, and the process was very easy. In any given city or town there were many tiny manufacturing concerns. Quality was another issue.

COLGATE AND COMPANY

But the man who exposed the hypocrisy was. Because DeRobigne Mortimer Bennett, National Liberal League member and editor of the Truth Seeker *(the first publication exposing Colgate's contraceptive claims), published freethinker Ezra Heywood's essay "Cupid's Yokes," which pointed out the foibles of marriage—and described Comstock as a "religio-monomaniac"—he received thirteen months hard labor. Colgate got richer.*

cuted: Comstock went after the little guys only, but they could be hard to catch.

Some of the big producers like Goodyear and other rubber manufacturers did remain, nominally, in the condom-making business *legally*. Though not at the pre-Comstock level, the major producers of rubbers took advantage of a loophole in the Comstock Act that allowed doctors to prescribe condoms for medical purposes. Any "extras" the rubber makers found themselves with were quietly sold to the same pharmacies that dispensed the legal condoms, as well as retailers who were not actually pharmacists but "druggist suppliers." Typically, these retailers simply placed the items in the rear of their stores, or behind the counter; word of mouth led customers into the condom outlets, where they would request their rubber goods, pay their bill, and exit with a small brown package under their arms.

On the rare occasion that the law did catch up with mass-

THE LITTLE GUYS

Morris Glattstine, a Polish Jew who purchased condoms from the big manufacturers to resell from his druggist supply store in Brooklyn, was one of those small entrepreneurs who was prosecuted by Comstock. In spite of being exposed by the free-thinkers, instead of Colgate being prosecuted for his birth control advertising, it was people like Glattstine who took the heat. The big manufacturers? Comstock never made a move against them.

WORLD EXPOSITION OF 1876

The mini rubber, or glans, condom (which fit just the head of the penis) was displayed at the World Expo-sition of Philadelphia in 1876, just a few years after the passing of the Comstock Act. Its German manu-facturers thought the device was a potentially prof-itable one, and by the turn of the twentieth century Germany was making some of the finest rubbers in the world.

produced rubbers, it was the small retailer who purchased and sold only small-job lots who took the heat. None of the big boys, like Goodyear and Goodrich, were charged or fined—or prevented from making their *medicinal* condoms. Their political connec-tions and the lobbying power worked not only to keep them in the business but also made sure no small-timers ever gained a foothold in the lucrative medicinal market.

⊰⊱⊰⊱⊰

No matter who was and was not caught, the condom industry thrived through both mail-order and bricks-and-mortar retail, as well as backdoor sales. Those who sold them via the mail were vulnerable because that is where Comstock's postal agents were most likely to catch them: but these distributors were all over the country and usually managed to allude the law or get away with minor fines. They were also remarkably resilient and cre-ative in the way they advertised and concealed their own identities. Condom advertising pseudonyms included terms like "Comstock Capotes," making clever use of the fanatic antisex crusader's name to iden-tify a birth control device. The advertisers themselves were careful to use creative titles when they advertised their goods and services in the circulars, newspapers, and penny pamphlets that could be found on any street corner in cities and towns. Especially popular with women and men selling their

USE IT AGAIN . . . OR NOT??

There was a lot of misunderstanding regarding just when and if the sheath was reusable. The manufacturers did not help resolve the confusion; some sold their wares individually, packaged in fancy boxes or elegant sets, often promising their products did not deteriorate and would "never need replacing." This left consumers wondering if that meant reusability or a long shelf life. Others were sold in larger quantities, cheaply packaged, and of such poor quality, reusing them would have been folly.

wares was the title "Madame." And the quantities many of the condom dealers dealt in was staggering. When German immigrant Joseph Backrach, who both produced and sold them, was caught by a Comstock agent, he had more than eleven thousand caps and condoms in stock. After Backrach paid his fine, he went right back to business.

It is not possible to know who produced their own and who were middlemen for producers or importers. It is certain that European animal intestines remained the most popular material for the manufacture of high-quality skin condoms; after 1870, between $35,000 and $50,000 a year was still being spent importing intestines into the United States for condom production.

CLASSES OF WOMEN

Although Comstock had driven the sex experts underground, he was not able to slow the unsinkable Mrs. Dr. Sarah Chase from continuing in the fine tradition of sex lecturers at the lyceum or from providing one-on-one services to women, including educating about condom use and even performing abortions. Chase was the Comstock era's most successful condom saleswoman. However, she was more than just a peddler; she was definitely of the spirit of her earlier counterpart, the Quaker sex lecturer Mary Gove.

Chase was a bona fide homeopath and a card-carrying feminist who gave lectures on the public circuit and at New York City's Cooper Union Academy from the 1870s into the twentieth century. Like Gove, she sold contraceptives after each of her lectures. But Gove had not had to deal with the likes of Anthony Comstock. When he discovered Chase was not only teaching about contraception but also selling condoms and other contraceptives after her speeches and through the mail, he was sure he had found his latest victim.

In spite of her activities, which included at least five arrests, Chase was one of those who Comstock could not get a judge or jury to convict; this was in spite of his attempt to illegally indict Chase, an effort that prompted her to file a ten-thousand-dollar lawsuit against him, claiming false arrest. Like others Comstock harassed, Sarah Chase managed to continue in the condom business for many years, and numbered as one of Comstock's bitterest failures.

MRS. DR. SARAH CHASE

The feminist homeopath was ahead of her times in many ways, but was also a product of her era. A member in good standing of the Institute of Heredity, Chase hypothesized that there were four "classes" of women, a circumstance dictated by heredity. At one of her many public lectures she told the packed audience of men and women that 30 percent of women were in class one, and all could and would make good wives. Class two consisted of 25 percent of all women, who made good wives but not good mothers; and class three, 20 percent of women, were good mothers but not good wives. She explained that it was unreasonable to expect one group to fulfill the duties of another and that a class-one woman had to be a "good animal" to survive the experience, a statement that peaked the audience's interest.

It was the women who applauded wildly though when Chase explained that there was a fourth class of women and that this group was definitely not fit to be mothers or wives. Rather, the "Old Maids" were the "thinkers, logicians, writers," the "teachers, dressmakers, physicians, artists, and lawyers." But the greatest applause came when Chase stated that she "honored . . . the woman who wouldn't palm herself off on a man when she knew she was unable to make either a wife or a mother. If a man wanted to improve his stock he wanted to marry the 3rd class of woman!"

The hundreds, possibly thousands, of women entrepreneurs in the condom business, all happily defying Comstock, were in it for the money. By the end of the nineteenth century, however, there were new faces in the battles over condom use, and they had nothing to do with production and sales. Birth control (a new phrase coined by America's most public birth control advocate) had become a part of the growing feminist agenda, and along with the struggle to get the right to vote, many feminists believed equality could not be achieved without the ability—the legal ability—to control the number of children women had. And it is here that the feminists and the condom often clashed.

Some early feminists approved of and even promoted its use as a simple, inexpensive way to prevent pregnancy. However, as the century moved forward and the feminist movement matured, more and more of its leaders reversed that stance and became very anticondom. They equated its use with the substandard rights of women, another example of something controlled by and decided upon by men, leaving women out of the decision-making process. Feminists preferred the diaphragm and spermicidal douches because those methods were strictly controlled by women.

ENTER MARGARET SANGER

America's premier birth control pioneer had mixed emotions about the condom. Margaret Sanger had begun her career as a birth control advocate while working as a nurse in New York City. Appalled at the living conditions of poor immigrant women in neighborhoods

MADAME RESTELL

One of Comstock's greatest personal victories was the arrest of Madame Restell, considered New York's most successful provider of birth control and "abortionist." Restell, born Ann Trow in Gloucestershire, England, had married a butcher and the pair immigrated to New York, where her husband died shortly after. She remarried a German-Russian immigrant, who was a freethinker involved with men like Robert Dale Owen and Charles Knowlton. Although she made a tidy income in her profession—and no doubt understood condom production through her first husband's experience as a butcher—Restell believed her work was important to other women. In order to entrap her, Comstock pretended to be a father with too many children to feed and went to Restell's beautiful mansion on Fifth Avenue in New York begging for birth control. She obliged by selling him a box of condoms and Comstock arrested the sixty-seven-year-old; Madame Restell was so horrified at the idea of being dragged through the courts and the gutter press (she had become popular fodder for yellow journalists like Horace Greeley), she committed suicide while bathing in the luxurious bathroom of her mansion rather than be put through the ordeal. The evidence against her? Comstock's men had searched her home and office and among other things they found were "ten dozen boxes of skins."

like the Tenderloin and Hell's Kitchen, she believed that the already terrible conditions in those areas of the city were made worse by having too many children. Sanger wrote treatises on the subject of birth control, including using condoms, and it was her attempt to send her tracts through the mail that got her into trouble with Comstock, who managed to put her in jail more than once during her long career as an activist.

Twice Sanger narrowly escaped Comstock's attempts to arrest her by escaping to Europe, where she learned more about birth control methods. While there, she increasingly adopted the European feminists' point of view, coming to believe as they did that the condom took control away from women, and she became concerned from a practical point of view that they did not offer the kind of protection she felt women deserved.

Eventually Sanger returned to open a birth control clinic in New York, modeled after that of Dutch doctor Aletta Jacobs. Shortly after opening her doors, however, Sanger was snagged again by Comstock, who shut down her efforts as "obscene." Ironically, after numerous setbacks due to Comstock's efforts to prevent her from educating poor women about birth control, it was during Sanger's last trial (actually her husband's, who had been arrested for trying to help the cause) that Comstock was finally taken out of the fight. While testifying during the 1915 trial, Comstock, now in his seventies, caught a chill in the drafty courtroom and died from complications soon after.

At that point, Comstockery had been in its death throes for some time, helped by determined advocates like Sanger, and the tidal wave of people who simply wanted to practice birth control—and an increasingly cynical public, who by the turn of the century thought Comstock was little more than an annoying throwback to the misplaced morality movement of an earlier time.

Although the condom had been a device traditionally used by middle-class white Americans, with the help of advocates like Sanger, immigrants who had not known about or had not had access to birth control were increasingly using many methods, including the condom. In addition, by the 1890s, it had also gained great favor among urban African Americans, with mail-order businesses advertising *French male safes* and *rubber articles* in popular African American magazines and newspapers. Even W. E. B. Du Bois favored the use of contraceptives as a way to control family size, which he believed promoted quality of life for the black family.

OUT WITH THE OLD AND IN WITH THE NEW . . .
AMERICANS AND COMSTOCK'S CONDOM LEGACY

By 1900, Anthony Comstock had confiscated 64,836 "articles for immoral use, of rubber, etc." His dedication may have pushed condom sales underground, but with or without him, the trade continued to flourish. The portability and profitability promoted their popularity, as the industry thrived in a kind of microeconomy: rubber and skin condoms could be produced in the home or tiny makeshift factories with little expense, unskilled labor, and nominal equipment. That fact also means that it is impossible to know how many condoms were being made, bought, sold, and used at this time; exact numbers do not become available until the mass production of latex condoms in the 1920s, when the condom went to Wall Street. But there is no doubt that condoms were everywhere.

THE HORATIO ALGER OF CONDOMS—
PORTRAIT OF A CONDOM TYCOON

Born to impoverished parents in southern Germany in 1865, Julius Schmidt began life with multiple challenges: he was born with a severely deformed leg and he was Jewish. But in his late teens, and with the help of his grandfather who was convinced American streets were paved with gold, Schmidt raised enough money for passage to New York. His ship docked in New York Harbor in 1882, and he arrived with nothing but his clothes and faith that he would succeed.

But poor Schmidt, instead of a magical world and instant wealth, he found himself in a crowded, dirty, and dangerous city, just another desperate immigrant. He also realized what so many who had come before him had: it was tough to make it in the New World.

Unable to find work, Schmidt had to sell his extra clothes in order to eat. But just as he was giving into fear and desperation, he landed a job cleaning animal intestines in a sausage-casing factory. And like the sausage makers and slaughterhouse workers of old, while performing this unpleasant job, the new German immigrant figured out the *other* use for the leftover bits of intestine it was his job to clean.

Julius Schmidt started his condom-making business in his home and then expanded by peddling his wares in the Tenderloin district—Comstock's original stomping ground—where brothels did a booming business and customers were happy to pay for the convenience.

Unfortunately for Schmidt, the Comstock Act of 1872 made his trade illegal. In 1890 it was Anthony Comstock himself who raided Schmidt's home on Manhattan's Forty-sixth Street, where he found almost seven hundred "articles to prevent contraception" along with the materials to make more. It was a sad sight to see the menacing Comstock, so tall and stout, pushing the diminutive Schmidt—who had to walk with crutches—out to the horse-drawn paddy wagon. Schmidt was arrested and had to be bailed out of jail. He also had to pay a fifty-dollar fine, a surprisingly low amount considering his heinous crime. But he was doing very well with his business, and Schmidt was not going to let a little bump in the condom road stop him from pursuing his life's work: the pursuit of wealth.

Although many of the city's condoms came from Europe, they were expensive; Schmidt had realized early on that men and women like himself were providing skins to those who could not afford the more expensive European brands.

Schmidt never let Comstock stop him from making and selling condoms and he continued to prosper, eventually naming his business Julius Schmid, Inc.—he dropped the *t*, believing it made him appear "less Jewish." He did so well, in fact, that he could afford to get married. American Elizabeth Wolf became Mrs. Schmid in 1892; she already had two sons and she and Julius had two more boys by 1898. When they were older, both Carl and Julius Schmid Jr. were instrumental in helping their father's business prosper well into the twentieth century.

Of course, even as the twentieth century dawned, the dissemination of anything contraceptive—whether it was how-to's or devices—was still illegal, so Schmid (along with many others) continued to be an underground producer of illegal contraband. He was so mindful of the need to keep his business a secret, Schmid stated on the 1900 national census that he was a "cap manufacturer"—a cute play on words since *cap* was the common term for a bottle stopper, but was also a post–Civil War euphemism for the condom.

By the time it was legal to produce condoms, Schmid had branched out into the rubber business and made a wide variety of rubber-based products. His advanced manufacturing methods had been developed in Germany, and the Schmids were the first in the United States to use them. Also a first, Schmid genuinely believed his condoms were the best quality available and he proved it by having them tested—remember the little problem with holes? He charged more for his brands but wanted his products to be the finest on the market, guaranteeing his were free from defects. He had come a long way from the early days.

Fortunately for Julius and the other condom manufacturers who by World War I were coming out of the condom closet—though it was still illegal to produce them—the Comstock Act was fading, and was finally revoked by the end of World War I. Better yet, at least from Schmid's perspective, Germany had been Europe's number one supplier of condoms prior to 1914, but war had virtually isolated Germany from the European economy, effectually stopping German export. Schmid had foreseen this possibility and had positioned himself to become the number one American exporter of condoms to the Allies, thus making an already successful entrepreneur a very rich man indeed.

In 1932, Schmid returned to his native Germany and purchased a German state-of-the-art rubber-manufacturing plant. Rather than try to run the plant from a distance, he made the decision to dismantle it, and shipped all of the equipment to New Jersey, reopening the German plant in the United States. As a Jew, his timing showed an amazing prescience: he barely missed Kristallnacht and the beginning of the Nazi destruction of all Jewish-owned businesses.

Despite the Depression, Schmid's company remained incredibly profitable and he died a very very rich man with a condom business that spanned the entire globe. His leading brands, Sheiks and Ramses, remained on the shelves until the late 1990s.

Julius Schmid was not the only immigrant who thrived in the shadowy world of condom production. The fact that the major rubber manufac-

THE LIBERAL LEAGUE

In 1877, in an attempt to dislodge Comstock from power, the Liberal League of Washington, DC, began a petition, originated by a bookstore owner in the capital, against Comstock and his appointment as special agent for the postal service. The petition was signed by what the Washington Post newspaper described as "a vast array of names. Among those already down in black and white are numbers of prominent publishers of New York, physicians and judges of note . . . photographers, printers, paper dealers, manufacturers, druggists and artists are also on the list."

It is perhaps surprising that, rather than complain first about his flagrant attempts to entrap his victims, the league chose to begin its complaint against Comstock with the argument that he was motivated to arrest innocent people because as special agent he "receives a salary of several thousand dollars per annum, and $2500 as mileage and extras," which acted as "incentives" to pursue the innocent. Calling Comstock a "peripatetic conservator of morals," they also brought up one of his stranger abuses of the office: he had had D. M. Bennett, a New York publisher and editor who had reprinted a pamphlet called an Open Letter to Jesus Christ, arrested for blasphemy—an offense not mentioned in the Comstock Act. Although the attempt to get rid of Comstock was admirable, given all of Comstock's "political ears," for some reason the process lost momentum and never made it to Congress. Instead, it took years of individual court decisions to slowly dismantle the dreaded act.

turers did not take the chance of making condoms their primary business—and could not have, since the skin condom remained the most popular type until the invention of latex— left a huge market open to those who were not welcome or even allowed into mainstream American businesses. A disproportionate number of condom manufacturers (and salesmen) were women, Jews, and immigrants, proving that little had really changed in this ancient business. They found an excellent niche for their illegal products and profited from the displaced prejudice, a prejudice especially evident in Anthony Comstock and his ilk.

CONFUSION, COMSTOCKERY, AND THE COURTS

Although it would take another twenty years to be overturned, the Comstock Act had lost a lot of its impact by the end of the nineteenth century. Sarah Chase's case was just one of many illustrating the fact that there were many judges and juries who felt Comstock was not just eccentric in his efforts to bring the law to bare against sinners; they hated his courtroom histrionics and were deeply concerned about the illegal tactics (entrapment) Comstock and his men so commonly used to root out condom merchants as well as other birth control providers. There were also a number of Supreme Court decisions that held that mail was a private matter, protected under the First and Fourth Amendments of the Constitution. These set limits on some of the tactics Comstock could employ to catch and prosecute mail-order condom businesses.

Even President Grant, who had entered into the presidency on the eve of the passing of the Comstock Act, ended up pardoning a number of those arrested and convicted under it. Most of them were condom dealers. Following Grant's lead, President Hayes also pardoned one of Comstock's victims. Ezra Heywood was a freethinker who had made fun of Comstock's efforts in a poetic "reflection on marriage," which got him arrested and sentenced to hard labor for his puns. He was freed by Hayes, who agreed with some judges and former president Grant: Comstock had simply gone too far.

PORTRAIT OF A COUPLE

Even at the height of the Comstock era, letters exchanged between women friends, sisters, and between husbands and wives illumine just how popular sheaths remained.

In the 1870s Daisy and Elmer of Baltimore exchanged frank letters about her desire to remain childless: Daisy did not want to be pregnant—ever—and asked her husband to do something to ensure she did not. Elmer's job required a lot of travel—hence the letters—and he obliged his wife by buying skins as he worked and passed through cities like Richmond and New Orleans. Daisy documented the ease by which her husband was able to buy the items and the casual nature of the purchases, along with his knowledge of the device.

But what really kept the condom market going and growing throughout this confused century? It was not court decisions and presidential pardons; it was the daily reality of men and women who simply needed or wanted to control their own destinies by controlling their own reproduction. In spite of that fact though, Comstock did have an impact on American society. His efforts drove the fledgling movement for public discussion of sex underground. Individuals continued to try to dictate their own sexual destinies, but the late nineteenth and early twentieth centuries are remembered for their odd combination of sexual experimentation, inhibition, and ignorance. Possibly the most dramatic and painful legacy of that ignorance is that as the second half of the nineteenth century progressed, the incidence of venereal infection skyrocketed.

Although the pox and the clap had long been a problem in places like late eighteenth-century Philadelphia, it was not until the latter half of the century that the spread of disease became an enormous, mostly silent, and untreated health problem, especially in the cities. The nineteenth-century condom was a birth control device, and its use as a disease preventative was limited. And though the oldest profession continued to thrive in cities and towns around the country, there was a code of silence that had been stamped onto the American sexual psyche by Comstockery; those who participated in prostitution simply took their chances.

This ignorance had a powerful impact on Americans. And it would take a terrible toll after the turn of the century, especially when the nation entered into the Great War.

NINE

obscenity laws, american tips, and french ticklers

WAS THERE AN ENGLISH COMSTOCK?

The second half of the nineteenth century was in many ways a thrilling period for English and European culture. Dickens, Eliot, and Hardy celebrated and castigated their own times; Wagner, Verdi, Brahms, and Strauss entertained larger and larger audiences with their ingenious works; and the great minds of the modern sciences like Darwin and Mendel were shocking the world with their observations about life on earth. By the 1870s, photography, the telegraph, the telephone, along with other amazing inventions and innovations reflected an increasingly technological world. But while great minds explored the new and the far reaching, the old struggles over right and wrong, moral versus immoral, and the human spirit versus "law and order" continued to vie for prominence, especially in the legal and political realms.

Under the guise of preventing vice from poisoning European society, but more likely with a view to peeking behind closed doors, specifically bedroom doors, beginning in the 1850s legislators throughout Europe were passing laws directed toward legislating sex. These ranged from outright bans on the sale of birth control devices to the more Comstockian-style statutes intended to prevent innocent citizens from being irrevocably harmed through exposure to smut.

Like Americans, Europeans tended to work around the laws, an easier task for them though, since there were no Señor, Monsieur, or Herr Comstocks to contend with. But some of the attempts to protect citizens from themselves, specifically those in Britain, did make life a little uncomfortable for the humble little condom.

In 1857, England's Lord Chief Justice Campbell introduced into the House of Lords the Obscene Publications Act, a bill the chief justice declared would stop the sale of the kind of written material that led to the corruption of the morals of innocent children, women, and the "weak of mind." Or, as Campbell declared dramatically, an act of law that would prevent the "sale of poison more deadly than prussic acid, strychnine or arsenic." He also benignly assured his fellow members of Parliament that his bill would *not* impede "*real* literary pursuits."

The first official to enforce the English antiobscenity law was a royal magistrate by the name of Hicklin. Being the first, Magistrate Hicklin had no precedents to follow, which allowed him to interpret the act according to his own conservative agenda. Although the law was intended to prevent sales or exchanges of pornographic materials, it had also been designed to protect the civil rights of Englishmen, shielding citizens from illegal search and seizure. Specifically, it stated that without a search warrant, no member of the constabulary could simply enter private property to look for obscene literature. Hicklin, however, chose to interpret this to mean that a search warrant could be issued on sworn information given by *anyone* who stated that an individual possessed pornographic publications intended for sale or distribution. *His* interpretation put the accused in the position of having to show cause as to why the authorities should not destroy the offending literature—and not arrest him. According to Hicklin then, the burden of proof fell to the owner of "obscene material," not the person making the charge.

Some British historians believe the Hicklin Act, as it came to be called, was the inspiration for the Comstock Act. Like the Comstock Act's effect on America's sex life, instead of the Hicklin Act keeping innocents free from smut, it did help drive Britain's sex trade underground, where it thrived throughout the last quarter of the nineteenth century. It did not, however, empower any one government agency or individual to persecute and prosecute in the way the Comstock Act had, leaving it up to individual police departments to enforce. Rather than Hicklin inspiring the Comstock Act, it was probably the Comstock Act that influenced a later English antiobscenity law, passed by the House of Lords in 1889, which certainly brought the British condom under official scrutiny.

THE "INDECENT ACT"

The Indecent Advertisements Act was one legislator's response to the tremendous number of ads popping up in British newspapers that touted an endless variety of cures for venereal disease; as in the United States, by the 1880s the pox was back in a big way in the United Kingdom. On the street, from storefronts, and through print advertising, quacks and charlatans hawked bogus cures to desperate victims.

The sponsor of the indecency act, the Earl of Meath, was a Christian philanthropist who to his credit had done a great deal of public good for London's poor. He supported organizations that advocated for the education of working-class boys, introduced physical education into the English school curriculum, and was a tireless advocate for setting aside green space for public parks. But for reasons known only to himself, Meath had an absolute horror of syphilis, believing any discussion, private or public, about its prevention or cure was obscene. No wonder he was so offended by the advertisements for curatives and preventatives plastered all over the city's cheap newspapers and broadsides. Meath wanted all of it banned as "detrimental to common decency."

The advertisements act, though vaguely worded, was intended to enable the judiciary to take legal action "against persons who advertise their specifics against a certain class of diseases of a nameless character" and pointedly included the "filthy advertisement of condoms." Instead of separating disease prevention from the cures offered by shysters taking advantage of desperate syphilitics, the act lumped cures and preventatives together, proving not only a misplaced prudery that had increasingly become the norm among late-century upper-crust "Victorians" but that actually ended up promoting sexual ignorance.

Even the royal family did not go unscathed by the growing cloak of sexual silence and its regrettable results. Unwilling to acknowledge the fact that her son had syphilis and help him seek proper treatment, Queen Victoria preferred to pretend it simply did not exist. As far as she and other family members were concerned, Victoria's son Prince Alfred, Duke of Edinburgh, had contracted a "mysterious malady." The Duke's son, Prince Alfred II, was also a victim of syphilis, but this time, to avoid further scandal, the lesser prince was exiled to Romania, where he died suffering from the dementia common to victims who went untreated. If only those royals had known about, and used, condoms.

The Indecent Advertisements Act certainly reflects the narrow-minded, dangerously naive mind-set of some late-century Englishmen, but in spite of the similarities between the English legislation and the Comstock Act, there were huge differences between the English and the American laws; the English laws were not utilized to *prevent* the sale of condoms, just their advertisement (and at that they were not successful), a kind of out-of-sight, out-of-mind approach by moralists who despised the condom as a physical representation of indecent behaviors.

No one went to jail for making, selling, or using them.

A PORTRAIT OF THE QUEEN

Queen Victoria may have been unwilling to admit to her family's problems with the clap, but that did not prevent her visage from being used by makers of the little device that might have saved her son's and grandson's lives. By the time of Queen Victoria's 1897 diamond jubilee, droll manufacturers produced very artistic condoms; they had the queen's portrait printed on them. For the more politically minded, there were also nicely made French letters with English prime minister Gladstone's image stamped on them.

These patriotic condoms were proudly sold in small gift shops along London's Petticoat Lane.

THE MARKET SIDE OF PROTECTION

Coyly referring to a quick trip to the chemist's for a supply of condoms, the expression "a little something for the weekend" was an English phrase that was coined at the time, and another example of the condom's lyrical influence on linguistics, and its common usage.

Just as they had been doing for hundreds of years, lots of small-time makers, working out of back rooms, butcher shops, and small storefronts, continued to produce a wide variety (and widely differing qualities) of condoms through to the end of the nineteenth century. England's first major *public* condom manufacturer, E. Lambert and Son of Dalston, opened in the 1870s; although Lambert's was the largest English manufacturer, the production of condoms was not limited to one company. There were a surprising number of brick-and-mortar businesses establishing in and around London and other major cities, and many of them did a very brisk business selling a wide variety of "little somethings for the weekend," as demonstrated by this somewhat remarkable exchange.

W. George was informed by the local council that he had to relocate his contraception business because of an 1897 urban renewal act demanding areas of London's Strand be redeveloped. His business, which he had opened in the early 1870s, was located on the busy Holywell Street in London. But W. George objected to the gross undervaluing of his business when it came time for the council to reimburse him for the loss of his property. By his estimation, his condom business was worth many thousands of pounds per annum (adjusting for inflation, that would be in the millions today), but the Government Board Valuer placed the business's worth (incorrectly) at only five hundred pounds. Undaunted, W. George pursued his case and hired a lawyer. As the representatives from both sides sat opposite one another in the council chambers, it leaves the reader wondering which of the two men was more embarrassed by the exchange.

The law required that anyone objecting to a government evaluation of

W. GEORGE VERSUS URBAN RENEWAL

Although he failed to prove his case to the hard-hearted government board valuer, Mr. Harrison's lawyer was eloquent in his argument for the inherent value of the Holywell Street location: ". . . this particular class of trade carried on, a trade for which the premises in their present position are best adapted. The very fact that Holywell Street is not a traffic thoroughfare, the very fact that people can go down Holywell Street and buy what they wish without being seen as much as they would be if they went into some handsome shop in the Strand, occupying a commanding position, is a fact which brings people to the shop, and that makes the shop more valuable because more trade is done thereby." The valuer disagreed and the case dragged on through 1901.

his business or property be allowed to mount a challenge of the proposed amount offered at a formal hearing. As W. George's hearing began, and already knowing the answer to the question, the council's muttonchopped solicitor began the formal questioning by asking W. George's legal representative just "What is the business done at this shop?" The lawyer answered vaguely that "general medical appliances" were sold there.

Almost whispering, the council solicitor asked, "Anything else?" After some hemming and hawing, W. George's rep replied that the "Claimant" sold "*American instruments . . . French letters . . . Spanish* and other *letters . . .*"

The answer seemed to help the council solicitor find his voice. He asked just who shopped at W. George's, to which the representative answered: "I think we are all gentlemen here, we all know about that, it is not secret. . . . They are almost a necessity nowadays— someone must sell them. . . . I may say that judges and clergymen, I know it for a fact, do use *letters*. . . . This class of business has to be carried on somewhere . . . yes, all respectable chemists sell them."

Not only does the unique exchange continue to illumine the use of condoms, but proves that they continued to acquire creative euphemisms as the years passed (and, as there is no mention of *Teutonic letters*, Englishmen apparently did not realize that by the end of the century many of their letters were actually imported from Germany, by then the number one supplier of rubbers for most of Europe). However, it also illustrates the continued hypocrisy surrounding condom use; when W. George took his case to a court of law, he tried in vain to force the council to understand how much his condom business netted. During the arguments, the government solicitor pompously urged the jury to find that the business "should be valued on a very different basis from a thoroughly respectable one." The High Bailiff was a little fairer, as he begrudgingly told the jury that they were to compensate the owner "fairly for the loss of his business, however unpleasant might be its character." In the end, the government recompensed W. George for less than 20 percent of his year of lost condom sales. There was no word on where the judges and clergymen would now purchase their *American instruments*.

Though disappointed about the loss of income, W. George (his real name was W. R. Harrison) did continue to do a thriving business through his mail-order catalog, where other suppliers as well as individuals could purchase *American Tips*, *Skin Letters* "available in two sizes, small and ordinary," and *Rubber Letters*, "the best, surest and most frequently used of any known appliance." He was in competition with barbers, chemists, surgical supply stores, pubs, and even tobacconists, as well as other mail-order businesses, but his was one of the best and highest-quality inventories in the business.

⧓

Perhaps one of the most innovative mail-order advertising campaigns in history appeared at this time. It was for "Rubber Goods for New Parents," appealing to couples who had just had babies. The rubber entrepreneurs checked birth announcements in local and national papers, then sent each couple a flyer explaining the benefits of their particular condoms, which were "foolproof" birth control. The upshot of the ads was to appeal to new parents who not only missed having sex but did not want to risk having another little darling. It was a very successful campaign.

⧓

The English had their anticondom critics, but no Englishman ever went so far as to try to legislate or prosecute in the American manner. The acts of the last half of the nineteenth century never produced a fanatic like Anthony Comstock, and legal actions against individuals were reserved mostly for high-visibility proponents of sex and disease education, free love, and those who sought to bring homosexuality out of the closet. The English birth control movement did meet with legal battles and legal resistance throughout the latter half of the nineteenth century. Its proponents and their leaders faced jail time if they were caught publishing and distributing literature written to educate about or promote birth control. But, not unlike Americans, the English—especially the middle class—purchased their condoms in ever-increasing numbers. The difference was that English law never made the selling or use of birth control devices illegal.

OOO LA LA

Elsewhere in Europe, the condom did not come under the same kind of scrutiny as in the United States and England. In 1868 a French doctor publicly denounced condom use, equating it with masturbation, and generally condemned sex with "coit avec le condom," but he was probably not in the majority. Historically speaking, the French had in many ways been the most open about condom use: true or not, they had long been credited with inventing the baudruche. And it is the French who

ODIOUS NAPOLEONIC CAPS

In spite of the important role Frenchmen had played in making the little sheath acceptable, by the time it was being more and more openly discussed in England and America, the French were not quite so publicly enthusiastic. As early as 1821, Charles-Louis Cadet de Gassicourt (who had been Emperor Napoleon Bonaparte's *pharmacien ordinaire*) was very public in his objections to pharmacies selling "health caps" and "English redingotes." He felt it degrading to a place otherwise dedicated to "real medicine."

Another Frenchman, writing anonymously to a proponent of contraception, took delight in criticizing the English use of the condom: for they "will require the odious and unhealthy preliminary, called, moucher la Chandelle [snuffing the candle], or some gross mechanical precaution." He was apparently unaware that the French continued to enjoy their baudruches and Parisian condom businesses did a thriving international trade throughout the nineteenth century.

continued the "tradition" of manufacturing with a great deal of imagination, and no little humor, an entertaining variety of letters. In fact, the most famous nineteenth-century baudruche was created by the French and is still around today.

The *French tickler* began life as a "serious" rubber condom, but with a little something extra, just for the ladies. The glass molds used for making ticklers were blown with little protuberances all around the outer walls, so that the finished rubber product came out with lots of fingers for "extra stimulation." The design was an attempt to get around the fifty-year-old complaint that rubbers were not comfortable, especially for women. But the clever French producers did not stop with the French tickler. By the 1890s, throughout Paris and other major city centers, a condom consumer could purchase any number of specialty baudruches that put the English prime minister's portrait to shame. These included *le porc-epic* (*the porcupine*), *l'inusable* (*hardwearing*), *le conquerant* (*the conqueror*), *le cocorico* (*the cock-a-doodle-do*), *le sainte-nitouche* (*the "she looks as if butter wouldn't melt in her mouth"*), and *le bibi chatouilleur* (*the baby tickler*)—definitely more interesting than sporting a portrait of Queen Victoria. And modern condoms really are humble in comparison.

NO TEUTONIC TICKLERS

Although the rest of Europe did not put the portraits of its royals or political leaders on condoms like the English, or show the astounding inventiveness of the French, they did continue to use them.

In late-century Germany, selling contraceptive devices was technically illegal, but because of lax legal enforcement, the strong desire to limit family size, and the German military's encouragement of disease prevention through condom use (which served to educate a lot of young men about its hows and whys), Germans knew about and used condoms extensively. They were also exposed to ads in their major newspapers, where advertisers employed obvious euphemisms like "rubber articles." And perhaps not surprisingly, German engineering was at its best when it came to condom production.

Rubber producers made their rubber skins from the most advanced manufacturing methods available, and by the turn of the century German rubbers were the highest quality and most popular in all of Europe. In fact, the Germans were not only supplying most European nations, they were also exporting to Australia, New Zealand, and Canada.

The Italians, on the other hand, were more inscrutable when it came to their use of condoms. Few population records were kept until 1861, when the Italian states unified as one nation. They also left very few personal records to help document just how large a role condom use played in fertility limitation. This is in part because of the tumultuous political upheaval of the second half of the nineteenth century and because of the influence of the Vatican. But mostly German-produced condoms were available from barbers and chemists in the major cities of Italy, and there are sufficient records available to make it clear that between 1800 and 1900, Italy had experienced a significant, and intentional, drop in fertility, and the condom played a role in that population decline. It was helpful, too, that though the sale of birth control devices was illegal in nineteenth-century Italy, condoms were sold as disease preventatives—common knowledge of their "other" use, of course, was just that. Unlike Americans and other Europeans, Italians had a long memory. They had, after all, "invented" the little device.

By the end of the century, the Dutch, along with the Swiss, Danes, and Swedes, bought German condoms and had their own small manufacturers of skins and rubbers; all were avid users of *condooms*.

In Holland, the first leader of the birth control movement there was also the first woman to graduate from a Dutch university and Holland's first woman doctor. Aletta Jacobs learned about contraception from the Germans and is credited with developing the first

AMSTERDAM'S BOSWELL

In the early 1890s, an anonymous tract titled My Secret Life *was published in Amsterdam. "Anonymous" sounds very much like fellow condom users from the prior century, as he moaned about his* French letters: "I was timid, used French letters, and took to carrying them in my purse again, but always hated them . . . I used to pay nine pence each . . . a sheath dulls enjoyment and if used frequently produces impotence in the man and disgust in both parties." He was more positive when he described "blowing up" a condom to use as a "dildo."*

diaphragm. She also approved of and recommended condoms, preferably made from silk. Whether or not these were widely available is unknown, but it is yet more evidence of the wide variety on the European market at the time, with the new rubbers vying with more traditional fabrics and guts that had been popular for many centuries, in many cultures.

One of the few places in Europe that remained stubbornly anticondom was Ireland. Although the Irish had suffered their first outbreak of the *English pox* in 1496, the condom had never been manufactured or sold—at least not legally—as disease prevention in that country. Not until the 1970s did the condom leave behind its sad history as foul contraband to quietly take its legal place—as a birth control device.

TEN

"the nineteenth century's greatest invention"

MUCKRAKERS, MORAL ARMOUR, AND THE GREAT WAR

As the nineteenth century came to a close, American Express had introduced traveler's checks, the term "spaceship" had come into use, and IBM was born—as the Tabulating Machine Company. H. G. Wells added to the new "outer space" genre with his Martians in *The War of the Worlds* and Conan Doyle introduced *The Adventures of Sherlock Holmes*. Suffragists on both sides of the pond were moving forward with their demands for the vote, some becoming martyrs to the cause. Telephones were all the rage and by 1891, Londoners could ring their friends in Paris; meanwhile, secretaries were tapping away on their 450,000 typewriters.

On the flip side, the negative effects of urbanization, immigration, and industrialization were being exposed by muckrakers like Jacob Riis and Upton Sinclair, who began a campaign to bring light to the horrible conditions many immigrants and child laborers in the United States endured. The British, meanwhile, were busy trying to keep their empire together. But for all the changes taking place during this period, some things remained constant: condoms were still the Western world's favorite birth control method.

SEX IN AMERICA

In a surprisingly candid lifestyle survey done in the 1890s by Celia Mosher, a woman doctor practicing in New York City, middle-class American women appear to have been very honest about their sex lives. Mosher found that the majority of women she canvassed reported a "healthy" enjoyment of sex, and that even those born before 1850 had consistently used birth control throughout their married lives—and many of them spoke specifically of using and even liking condoms. A decade later, another woman doctor conducted a similar survey and she found that, by 1900, the statistics remained the same and that 45 percent of her respondents used and appreciated condoms.

TEDDY'S TIRADES AND WILLFUL STERILITY

Unlike Grant and Hayes, and influenced by the tenets of social Darwinism, native-born middle-class men and women by the late nineteenth century were ranting against what came to be dubbed "racial suicide," meaning those WASPs who practiced fertility control. They claimed that these birth control users were forsaking their natural duties as American citizens. The fears were fueled by the massive immigration of the times, which meant that the white race was going to be outbred by the "other."

Leading the racial suicide charge in 1911 was the voluble and outspoken political leader and former president Theodore Roosevelt. In a speech he made about this, one of his favorite hobbyhorses, he said:

> *This UNITED STATES shares with other English-speaking countries the melancholy and discreditable position of coming next to the people of France, among great civilized countries, in that rapid decline of the birthrate which inevitably signalizes race decay, and which, if unchecked, means racial death. . . .*
>
> *The American stock is being cursed with the curse of sterility, and it is earning the curse, because the sterility is willful. It is due to moral, and not physiological, shortcomings. It is due to coldness, to selfishness, to love of ease, to shrinking from risk, to an utter and pitiful failure in sense of perspective and in power of weighing what really makes the highest joy, and to a rooting out of the sense of duty or a twisting of that sense into improper channels. . . .*
>
> *During the last decade the increase in population of the United States was almost two-thirds by immigration, the increase by birthrate showing a far lower percentage than ever before. . . .*

> *Again, to quiet their uneasy consciences, cheap and shallow men and women, when confronted with these facts, answer that "quality is better than quantity," and that decrease of numbers will mean increase in individual prosperity. It is false. When quantity falls off, thanks to willful sterility, the quality will go down too. We can say that, if the processes now at work for a generation continue to work in the same manner and at the same rate of increase during the present century, by its end France will not carry the weight in the civilized world that Belgium now does, and the English-speaking peoples will not carry anything like the weight that the Spanish-speaking peoples now do, and the future of the white race will rest in the hands of the German and the Slav. Are Americans really content that this land of promise, this land of the future, this abounding and vigorous nation, shall become decrepit in what ought to be the flower of its early manhood? Our forefathers were the heroes of the tremendous epic that tells of the conquest of a continent. The conquerors, the men who dared and did, with hearts of steel and thews [sinews] of iron, looked fearlessly into the eyes of the future, and quailed before no task and no danger; are their sons and daughters, in love of effortless ease and fear of all work and risk, to let the blood of the pioneers die out of the land because they shrink from the most elemental duties of manhood and womanhood? . . .*

But overall, the condom dichotomy remained the same through to the end of the century: on one hand, the Comstock Act would not be overturned until after World War I, so the condom had to remain in the closet, legally. On the other hand, the law was in direct conflict with the desire on the parts of so many to be in control of their own sexual destinies. And, where there was money to be made, there were always people willing to take their chances by flaunting the law and producing for a hungry market an ever-increasing variety of skins, capotes, and rubber goods.

In 1903 Teddy Roosevelt, America's first progressive president, took office and his presidency ushered in a time when vital public agencies were created to protect the health and well-being of Americans. Under the Progressive umbrella, the followers of people like Margaret Sanger pursued their goals of sexual, political, and social equality. However, as with the nineteenth, the reformers of the twentieth century did not make the direct connection between the condom and health, in spite of the soaring VD rate. Instead, there was an interesting mixture of prudish—moralistic—calls for abstinence and for education about sexually transmitted diseases, but nothing was said about "practical prevention."

As the nineteenth century ended, the use of rubbers continued to increase—but as birth control. Unlike the earlier history of the condom, when even aristocrats like Casanova were very careful to use protection to "save the fair sex from anxiety," it was not a notion that had stood the test of time, at least not in nineteenth- and early twentieth-century America. As the venereal disease rate climbed throughout the nineteenth century, the medical community and the moral watchdogs increasingly perceived sexually transmitted diseases as punishment for the sins of the sexually obsessed, leaving it to individual Americans to (re)discover the condom as a disease preventative.

MORAL PROPHYLAXIS

There should be taught such disgust and dread of these conditions that naught would induce the seeking of a polluted source for the sake of gratifying a controllable desire.

Into the first decades of the twentieth century, the prejudice against victims of venereal disease was so great that even large, well-equipped hospitals like Boston's Massachusetts General excluded all syphilitics. The same was true of hospitals throughout the country. For years, the American medical community simply sat on the fence, rarely speaking out about education and prevention.

Yet for all the fear and prejudice, and in spite of the lingering effects of the Comstock Act, America's sex trade was burgeoning. In 1900, Manhattan alone had at least fifteen thousand prostitutes plying their trade in the streets, working in brothels, back rooms of saloons, and even turning tricks in cafes. But this was a new age for reformers and a significant number of those who wanted to end the sex trade once and for all approached the problem quite differently from their nineteenth-century counterparts; for the first time, some reformers pointed out that men, not women, drove the trade, profiting by exploiting women as their pimps and as patrons. The reformers also recognized the relationship between the increase in prostitution and that of venereal disease, and they began the fight to bring the problem out of the closet and into the national spotlight.

Some state legislatures also got involved with the struggle against the spread of venereal disease by passing laws requiring physicians to report VD cases to the public health authorities. This, however, represented a dilemma for doctors, who rarely complied with the rules because they feared that it would lead to victims hiding their affliction. One physician was quoted as saying: "The treatment of venereal diseases has too long been left in the hands of charlatans and leeches who suck out the gold while they frighten their victims into silence." Another was more direct: "If physicians are required to report these patients by name, they will in short time, if they are honest, have no patients to report."

In spite of sporadic political attempts to deal with venereal outbreaks, as the Progressive Era matured, it was the social hygienists (so-called because they were determined to sanitize American sexual behaviors) who began the campaign to end public ignorance and misunderstanding about venereal diseases. This group was made up of reform-minded activists and medical experts and was the first organization in American history to recognize that the only way to end VD was to go public about its prevention.

The hygienists also made public something about VD that had been recognized only recently: science had proven that those who contracted syphilis were not the only victims. Many innocent wives and children suffered the long-term effects of the disease, because women could be infected by their husbands, and then give birth to children who suffered from the birth defects (and early deaths) common to babies born of syphilitics. The American Society for Sanitary and Moral Prophylaxis put it like this:

> Now the role of muck-raker is considered neither dignified nor desirable, the work of delving in the filth of human weakness and depravity is unsavory, even repulsive; it can be undertaken only from a sense of duty, but the muck is there and needs to be raked. . . . The public should know that

the introduction of venereal infection into marriage constitutes its chief social danger and at the same time makes up the saddest chapter in the martyrdom of women.

History, though, had proved time and again that prevention was not achieved just through pious declarations, and the hygienists, alas, were not interested in the condom.

> *I have spared no pains to make known that my plays are built to induce, not voluptuous reverie but intellectual interest, not romantic rhapsody but humane concern.*
> —George Bernard Shaw

SHAW'S ILLUMINATED GANGRENE

Letters were so popular in late nineteenth-century England that literary giant George Barnard Shaw boldly (and incorrectly) stated that the condom was the nineteenth century's "greatest invention." Shaw apparently had no idea of the history of the condom, but his exposure to England's pro-condom birth controllers had convinced him of their importance. Unlike the American social hygienist movement, England's version did have its condom adherents and they had a strange bedfellow in the famous—and often infamous—Irish playwright.

Shaw was very active in a number of the reform movements taking place in England in the late nineteenth century, marching hand-in-hand with birth control advocates like Betsy Besant and Marie Stopes as well as militant Irish freedom fighters. But Shaw's greatest contribution to the promotion of condom use—and to women's rights—was his play *Mrs. Warren's Profession*. In this terribly controversial work, Shaw tried to enlighten English and American audiences about the social reasons for prostitution and why women were often forced into the profession. He wrote *Mrs. Warren* to help both societies understand that prostitutes were not licentious sinners deserving to contract syphilis, as so many Victorians—and social hygienists—believed. Rather, he strove to convince the public that prostitution and the resulting spread of venereal disease was a product of the oppression of women, a belief he shared in common with some social reformers. Ultimately, he hoped to see an end to the trade, but in the meantime to at least educate women about "safe" sex. He also hoped to convince men to take the initiative and use sheaths.

But *Mrs. Warren's Profession* was slammed by American critics, as it had been by British, as "gross sensation," "wholly immoral and degenerate," and "illuminated gangrene." In 1905 it played only one night in a New York theater, after which Anthony Comstock himself had the entire cast arrested for indecency. Strangely, although *Mrs. Warren* was panned by critics and Comstock, it was resurrected later and actually performed in Washington, DC, for President Woodrow Wilson, America's third Progressive president, his cabinet members, and chosen congressmen, with the intention of educating them about how and why women became prostitutes.

Judging by what happened during World War I, Shaw's message was lost on this group of gentlemen.

> *The notion that Mrs. Warren must be a fiend is only an example of the violence and passion which the slightest reference to sex arouses in undisciplined minds, and which makes it seem natural for our lawgivers to punish silly and negligible indecencies with a ferocity unknown in dealing with, for example, ruinous financial swindling. Had my play been titled* Mr. Warren's Profession, *and* Mr. Warren *been a bookmaker, nobody would have expected me to make him a villain as well.*
>
> —Shaw's response to his critics

WITH THE LIGHTS TURNED OUT— SEX EDUCATION IN "PROGRESSIVE" AMERICA

In spite of the efforts of some of the more enlightened hygienists, this era was an odd mix of progressivism and leftover Victorian morals. Though it is during this time that "sex education," a new concept in public schooling, was born, the intention was to help clean up American sexual mores, not help the young understand themselves and their own sexuality. Courses and curriculum development were plagued with conflict within the movement itself over just how, when, and by whom the message of prevention should be delivered. The arguments, like those specifically about venereal disease prevention, began more than a hundred years ago, and they are still being debated today.

There were those who believed sex education belonged at home, which meant little more than remaining status quo—and at risk. Others believed only specially trained teachers (one of the positive outcomes of the Progressive movement was the development of specialized, university-based training for educators) should be allowed to teach such a delicate and important subject. It was not, however, necessarily a very open-minded curriculum.

Columbia University Teachers College, one of America's premier colleges for teachers, then as now, required teachers-in-training to attend classes in "sexual hygiene." One teacher-preparation manual explained that it was vital for new teachers to understand that students' daydreaming about sex was even worse than masturbation: daydreaming could go on and on . . . not so with masturbation. Other programs insisted that teachers know about and preach that abstinence was the only acceptable behavior, except when sex was necessary for procreation. Human nature did not influence the curriculum.

Oddly, in spite of the stilted and puritanical language used by the Progressives and medical experts in the first few decades of the twentieth century, with all the arguments and leftover prudery, the hygienists' conversations and debates did serve to bring VD education out into the open, and that was a step in the right direction. This fact, along with the demise of the Comstock Act in 1918, began to pave the way to making the condom at long last legitimate. But it took a world war, not the Progressive movement, to really bring the condom out into the light and back to its necessary role as a disease preventative.

FDR AND BLACK JACK

In 1916, while commanding troops along the unstable Mexican-American border, General Black Jack Pershing had the same concerns about his army that had supposedly led King Charles II of England to provide condoms to his men; VD was a huge problem among American soldiers and Pershing did not want his ranks to be decimated by the contagion. Black Jack proved to be a forward-thinking leader when he took it upon himself to try to prevent the growing problem of his soldiers contracting VD while visiting the many brothels that popped up wherever the men were stationed. He devised a system of army-controlled "clean" brothels, where condoms were provided when available and the women were "regulated" by army physicians. His efforts were rewarded with a decreased rate of VD and still-happy soldiers. And, Pershing was a politician first: he understood the sexually confused climate he was working in. He did not advertise his success.

> ## ORIGINS OF
> ## *PROPHYLACTIC*
> The term first appeared in writing in 1574 in a book discussing "Prophi-lacticke that preventeth diseases," a reference that stuck: prophylactic or prophylaxis *has always referred to preservation of health, both in people and in animals. The term was borrowed by military medicine, first as a reference to the creams used to prevent venereal disease, and eventually as a catch-all phrase, "preventative prophylactic" or "preventative prophylaxis," meaning a combination of condoms and creams issued to soldiers and sailors in hopes of preventing VD. It was a common condom euphemism by WWI.*

Meanwhile, there were a number of doctors in the American navy who had served on German ships in the first years of the twentieth century, and they had witnessed the trials and successes of the German navy's anti-VD program. The strategy was one of prevention (freely distributed *preservatifs*), early detection (a German innovation), and postexposure chemical treatment. (The French pioneered the antisyphilis drug Salvarsan, but its first successful testing was done in England at the Rochester Row Military Hospital in 1911. It was the Germans, however, who adopted its use for all of their military, making it, in a sense, a German medical breakthrough.) No German sailor went aboard ship without his "kit" and this remained true until World War II. The American naval physicians admired the Germans' practical, straightforward approach and took it upon themselves to put together anti-VD packets, which were provided to American sailors serving on ships in Asia. American army officials who saw the kits got into the act. In 1910, groups of soldiers were given supplies for VD prevention; this was actually a test to determine whether or not soldiers would even bother to use preventatives and if their use would impact the VD rate among the chosen groups of soldiers. The experiment was a huge success.

Assistant Secretary of the Navy Franklin Delano Roosevelt got very excited when he heard about the sailors' kits. FDR immediately ordered that all American sailors serving on ships overseas be supplied with what became known as *prophylaxis kits*. Although the word *prophylaxis* was intended to describe the entire process of prevention and cure, FDR's reference coined the latest euphemism for the condom. *Prophylaxis* was soon shortened to *pro*, which stuck through to the end of World War II.

FDR AND TEDDY

It is one of those strange twists of fate that distant cousins ended up being two of the most important American presidents of the twentieth century. But the coincidences between these two larger-than-life characters do not end there. As Teddy rose to prominence in the Republican Party in the late nineteenth century, he held any number of political positions, one being the assistant secretary of the navy. When his boss, the secretary, had taken the day off, Teddy managed to maneuver the United States into the Spanish-American War. A decade later, FDR also became the assistant secretary of the navy. Although his contribution to history while holding that office is not quite so spectacular, FDR, also taking advantage of his boss's absence, ordered that all sailors be issued "pro kits," laying the groundwork for military anti-VD policy for much of the twentieth century.

HISTORY REPEATS ITSELF—
THE FUNDAMENTAL CONDOM

The economically and politically powerful members of the social hygiene movement were furious when they found out about FDR's move, and they vetoed any future plans to supply members of the military with pros. These moral scions claimed that providing condoms to sailors and soldiers was like giving them a green light to "behave promiscuously." After all, bad behavior should be punished, not aided and abetted. The anti-prophylaxis hygienists had a powerful ally in Josephus Daniels.

Woodrow Wilson's new secretary of the navy, appointed just before America's entry into World War I, had been away on business the day his assistant, FDR, had ordered the naval prophylaxis kits. A fundamentalist Christian, Daniels believed VD was divine punishment for the sin of having sex for any purpose other than reproduction. It turned out that even before FDR got involved, quite a few commanders—aware of the "Asian" experiment and tired of losing valuable time and labor to disease—had also been putting together their own kits and selling them onboard their ships. They knew what VD did to the ranks and also knew preaching abstinence was a waste of breath.

Daniels's first act as secretary of the navy was to demand that the commanders stop selling these devices to their sailors and to put an end to Roosevelt's prophylaxis provisions:

> It is wicked to encourage and approve placing in the hands of the men an appliance which will lead them to think that they may indulge in practices which are not sanctioned by moral, military or civil law, with impunity, and the use of which would tend to subvert and destroy the very foundations of our moral and Christian beliefs and teachings in regard to these sexual matters.

It was in this muddled atmosphere that the United States made its late entry into Europe's Great War.

SLACKERS, SLUTS, AND SYPHILIS

The United States became involved in World War I in 1917, three years after it had begun. When Woodrow Wilson committed to sending troops to France, French prime minister Georges Clemenceau generously informed Wilson's secretary of war that the American expeditionary forces would have access to the French army's regulated brothels, where soldiers could visit "clean" prostitutes. This had been standard practice for the French military since Napoleon, and what better way to control the spread of syphilis among the troops? The American secretary's response to the translated message was, "Oh my God, don't tell the president or he'll pull out of this war before we send the first troops!"

Mystified by the negative response to his generous offer, and concerned about the ramifications of the American insistence that the French brothels be off limits to the doughboys (the greatest concern was that the Americans would go to *clandestines*—unregulated prostitutes—spreading syphilis as they went), as American troops began to arrive in France, Clemenceau had an inspector from the French surgeon general's office do an official study of the French military brothels. What the inspector concluded was that the American policies were prudish and repressive, ignoring the realities of the male libido: allowed

PUTES AND GERMANS

Perhaps such a thorough embracing of condoms had something to do with history. During the Franco-German War (1870–71), rumors of a French plan to infect German soldiers with venereal disease spread through the ranks. It was said that French putes were being recruited to infiltrate the ranks in order to lay waste to the German troops, with no shots fired. A play from the time helped perpetuate the rumor, one that reemerged during WWI: "Let us fall upon the German soldiers. We are monsters. Let us bare the brand through every street and beat the enemy from our fatherland!"

or not, as soon as they got off the boats American soldiers were making a beeline for the brothels. Interestingly, the inspector also revealed what had been intentionally hidden by the American military—American soldiers were bringing syphilis with them to France and infecting the French prostitutes they were not supposed to be consorting with. In his final report, the French inspector concluded that

> beginning with the principle that chastity is possible, they have declared an official continence; and they confide to religion and morals the duty of maintaining morality in man and keeping him always master of his passions. They depend, however, on violent exercise to afford distraction and to diminish the desire for their soldiers.

As the French inspector had found out, "violent exercise" did not work.

INVISIBLE PROPHYLAXIS

Despite Wilson's explicit and sexually charged letters to both of his wives, publicly he was a very pious and prim man. As illustrated by the secretary of the navy's attitudes, Wilson selected a staff that mirrored his own beliefs, and the American military was dominated by like-minded prudes. Secretary of War Newton Baker's words encapsulate the group's approach to protecting the American military from disease:

> These boys are going to France; they are going to face conditions we do not like to talk about, that we do not like to think about. . . . I want them armed; I want them adequately armed and clothed by their Government; but I want them to have invisible armor to take with them. I want them to have an armor made up of a set of social habits replacing those of their homes and communities . . . a moral and intellectual armor for their protection overseas.

WOODROW WILSON, A MAN OF LETTERS

Wilson may have been a self-proclaimed moralist and a public paragon of religious faith, but his personal life did not necessarily reflect that fact. Within a year of his first wife's death, he had remarried Edith Galt Wilson. To Edith, Wilson wrote torrid, sexually explicit love letters—both before and after marriage—leaving behind evidence of his having been one of America's "sexier" presidents.

To the Soldiers of the National Army

". . . . . Everything that you do will be watched with the deepest interest and with deepest solicitude, not only by those who are near and dear to you, but by the whole nation besides . . . The eyes of all the world will be upon you, because you are in some special sense the soldiers of freedom.

Let it be your pride, therefore, to show all men everywhere not only what good soldiers you are, but also what good men you are, keeping yourselves fit and straight in everything, and pure and clean through and through.

. . . . . My affectionate confidence goes with you in every battle and every test. God keep and guide you."

WOODROW WILSON.

The White House, Washington.

Lord Kitchener's Instructions to Soldiers

"It is discreditable, and even dishonest, that by contracting through self-indulgence a disease which he can avoid, a man should render himself incapable of doing that work for his country which he enlisted to do.

"Every man can by self-control restrain the indulgence of those imprudent and reckless impulses that so often lead men astray, and he who thus resists is a better soldier and a better man than the man of weaker will who allows his bodily appetites to rule him and who lacks the strength of character to resist temptation, and to refuse to follow any bad example he may see before him."

Woodrow Wilson and Lord Kitchener: Words to the troops

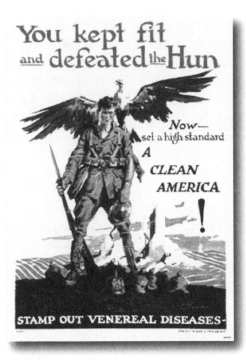

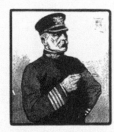

Surgeon Sage Says—

Only a poor boob pays his money, loses his watch, gets the syph, and brags that he's had a good time.

The French premier could have told him that this was not the armor the doughboys really needed.

Though there were many military surgeons and commanders who felt it was foolish and shortsighted not to supply real prophylaxis to their men, voices of reason were not heeded. Instead, sailors and soldiers were taught that the best way to prevent infection from venereal diseases was through abstinence. Drill sergeants and officers were ordered to provide soldiers with "invisible armor" rather than the practical sort. In lecturing the new recruits about abstinence, their leaders told them this about their penises: "Forget them, don't think about them, or dwell upon them. Live a good and vigorous life and they will take care of themselves."

"Only slackers consort with sluts which leads to syphilis," and "Live straight, so you can shoot straight," was the only help the American army was given. Not surprisingly, it did not work. Although the military—specifically the army—would not admit it, 70 percent of those soldiers infected with syphilis had actually gotten it stateside, from American prostitutes working at the many brothels just outside of the army posts where the new recruits were trained. Instead of facing this fact and fixing the problem, army officials blamed French prostitutes and warned the doughboys of the dangers of dalliances with French women. That, like all the other efforts to prevent men from getting the clap, failed.

America's great army was the only force in Europe not supplied with condoms as a standard part of their kit. Individual government officials, as well as organizations like the American Social Hygiene Association, fought tooth and nail to keep the condom out of the hands and off the penises of "our boys" in the military, and continued to cite such convincing arguments as: if you "risked" getting a venereal disease and caught one, then you deserved it. Not very progressive.

But all the pompous talk at home did not stop some American military men from procuring condoms from vendors selling them in and near the American "R and R" stations, as well as from the prostitutes who were routinely supplied by French officials, from barbers in the cities and towns—

and from other Allied soldiers, all of whom had access to a free and ready supply of American-made rubbers, sheaths, and French letters.

WERE THE ALLIES "CLEAN"?

Venereal disease and its prevention have never taken center stage in any Western history, but in those brief mentions of the VD problems of World War I, historians generally state that the English and French were well prepared with protection. Full stop. However, this is, in fact, far too simplistic, especially in regard to the English, who also suffered from the remnants of the prudish—and hypocritical—Victorian era.

First, as mentioned in previous chapters, there was never a limit or prohibition on the sales and marketing of condoms in the United Kingdom. But like the rest of the Western world, what was practiced in one arena was not always so in another. As late as 1914, the British military was still being subjected to the old sexual purity literature, where men were told that they should practice "cleanliness, moderation, pure air and self-control... avoiding impure conversation, thought and temptation." Lord Kitchener himself appealed to the British expeditionary force to "keep constantly on your guard against any excesses. In this new experience you may find temptations both in wine and women. You must entirely resist both temptations and while treating women with perfect courtesy, you should avoid any intimacy."

His was not an isolated prudishness from the old days. His words are very much a reflection of just how many military leaders approached

CLASS AND THE CONDOM

Especially early in the war, there was a defined difference between the information provided to English officers, who came from the upper classes, about venereal disease prevention, and that given to the poor and working-class soldiers. It was said that "the officers are better off" and "in comparative luxury, knowledge, and armour stand them in good stead." Whereas, the enlisted men had to make "the best of it in a thorny ditch" with any woman they could find ... without condoms. This in turn led many a soldier to find himself "standing in a queue later at the Red Lamp clinic," hoping for a cure after the fact. In 1917 the British military finally wised up.

the subject of sex and the soldier. But there was more than one school of thought on just how to keep the British military free of disease. When their men were not stuck in the foxholes at the front, some officers tried to occupy them with sports and recreation; this, in conjunction with extreme stigma if caught, was thought to be a good way to discourage licentious behaviors.

The stigma part of the philosophy included public censure of a sort. In the first few years of war, any British military member found to have a venereal disease at a clinic or at a "dangle parade"—those hated and embarrassing spot inspections of the private parts—was punished by having his family members notified of his illness. This draconian approach was ended in 1916 when an officer committed suicide after finding out his wife had been informed. After that, the family was simply told their loved one had been hospitalized—perhaps not a great improvement.

The treatments themselves may also have been enough of a punishment, since they could be painful and some had severe side effects, but even that did not deter individual soldiers from actually trying to get a case of the clap—anything not to return to the trenches. Some leaders believed in and tried the French model, which was to regulate prostitution, sanctioning only certain brothels in order to control disease. That did not work either.

Though too late for some, what did work well was a practical and scientific approach, one that did not rely on philosophy or self-restraint or waste medical personnel's time and energy—an *intelligent* (rather than moralistic) prophylaxis. Easy and unfettered access was the cheapest, safest, and most humane approach and the one that finally won out before the end of the Great War.

The English military eventually took its lead from one of the colonies.

Sexually speaking, the New Zealanders were the best equipped of any, with supplies of more condoms and postcoital treatment than their soldiers or sailors could possibly ever use. Australians were also routinely supplied with "blue light kits," as were the Canadians. Although British soldiers continued to contract VD (something some historians believe was very much a class-driven phenomenon), the numbers dropped tremendously when their military leaders routinely supplied their troops with rubbers; these even came in a variety of sizes (small, medium, or large), and colors (rose, drab, or ivory), with or without a "teat" end.

AXIS PROPHYLAXIS

The Allies were not the only ones familiar with condom use for disease prevention. The Axis military was provided with state-of-the-art German-made condoms throughout the war. Just as before the war, every German sailor and soldier had his own generous supply of *preservatifs*.

The Austrian military ran official brothels, and leaders were very cautious about making sure their facilities had official signs clearly posted with the rules of how and what the soldiers were to do when they used the services of the government-supplied prostitutes. These included directives for both the soldiers and the women, and were printed in German, Hungarian, and Croatian. The posts also made it clear that the girls were expected to reject "diseased guests," as well as make sure every man used a condom: "The girl should demand of the guest that he use a *preventative instrument*."

The brothels did not provide them for free, but each sign included a statement about cost: "*Preservatives* are available at the price of . . ." and the last line on the signs was one of advice: "The best-known protection against infection is the use of a condom which is to be drawn carefully over the member and then sufficiently lubricated with borated Vaseline." Businesslike, but very effective.

> ## NAPOLEON'S CONDOMS
> *One of Italy's most famous artists, military leaders, and lotharios, Gabriele D'Annunzio bragged about the fact that more than one thousand husbands hated him though he was careful to protect himself and his lovers; D'Annunzio had won Napoleon's snuff box in a bet and not only took his "lucky charm" with him into battle but also kept it filled with condoms.*

LOVE 'EM OR HATE 'EM . . .

The VD rate among American soldiers was very high. Military doctors and commanders found that, shortly after entering the war, orders or not, there were so many men already infected or at risk, they had to provide some kind of protection. This led to "prophylactic stations," where soldiers could go for treatment if they felt they might be at risk—but these were postcoital chemical treatments. In addition, the stations were difficult to provide, staff, and maintain, which led some commanders to quietly find ways to provide condoms to their men whenever possible—those commanders included Black Jack Pershing, who publicly denounced the condom, but privately recognized the need.

The narrow-minded, hypocritical approach to venereal disease protection and prevention—and lack thereof—took a terrible toll on the American fighting force. It led to a historically high incidence of syphilis and gonorrhea (almost 400,000 cases by the end of the war), which impacted military readiness, morale, and cost the American government a fortune in medical treatment. It was a tragedy that taught military leaders—and politicians— a painful lesson, and at least in this case, history would not repeat itself.

WAR COMMERCE

Condom magnet Julius Schmid's business was going strong in the 1910s. Ever the consummate businessman, as the winds of war began to blow, the native German recognized that the primary producer of European rubbers, Germany, would no longer be able to sell to other European nations. Schmid also knew of the European, Australian, and New Zealander militaries' policies on providing prophylaxis to their men. With this in mind, Schmid geared up to supply the European allies with condoms. It was a brilliant business strategy. Schmid's overseas sales boomed during the war, especially those to England, where by the end of the nineteenth century German rubbers had dominated the market but were no longer available because of the war.

Schmid was not alone in seeing wartime as a chance to expand his condom production and sales. Merle Youngs, founder of Youngs Rubber Company, saw a golden opportunity to pick up where the beleaguered English rubber industry had left off—and it was at this time that the most advanced—and most famous—condom was born: the first Trojans were produced in 1916.

But it was not just the foreign market Schmid was interested in; he was convinced that if Ramses, Sheiks, and Trojans teamed up, Schmid and Youngs could find a legitimate way to sell condoms to the American military, something Schmid felt would be too tall an order for just one manufacturer. In agreement that sales would skyrocket and both companies would make a fortune, the men directed their lawyer to send a letter to the US Secretary General, making sure not to mention the two of them by name or to identify the names of their companies. The lawyer inquired as to whether the secretary actually recommended, or was planning to recommend, "this kind" of disease-preventing prophylaxis to his military physicians. Interestingly, the letter was worded in such a way as to actually determine whether or not the official considered it legal to produce condoms (or *condrums*, a misspelling that may or may not have been a typo in the letter).

This backdoor approach to condom marketing was just a few years ahead of its time, and although their request was denied—in not-very-friendly language—the two condom producers still benefited from the fortunes of war.

COMSTOCKERY'S LAST GASP

Not long before the end of World War I, the 1918 Crane Act finally ended the legal ban on condom sales and production in the United States. Oddly, it was Margaret Sanger who inadvertently opened up the door to the legalization of condoms when she provided them at her short-lived birth control clinic in New York. She was arrested for her efforts and the case went to court. The first judge dismissed Sanger's claim that women not only had the right to use birth control, but it also was a social obligation, helping to alleviate poverty, overcrowding, and lessening the need for abortions, to mention a few of the reasons she gave. The judge, on the other hand, believed that women had no right to that "sort of regulation" and that sex was only for reproduction. But that did not stop Sanger; the second time the case went to court, the tide had finally turned and the abuses of the Comstock Act were ended at long last.

Influenced by the fact that American politicians and the medical profession had been forced to take the venereal disease epidemic (military and civilian) seriously, going so far as to create a division within the US Public Health Services (the Division of Venereal Diseases), and committing millions of dollars to irradiate the scourge, Judge Frederick Crane of the New York Court of Appeals permanently removed the legal limitations of selling, producing, or educating about condom use when he stated that condoms were disease preventatives. He also cited them as health aids because they prevented dangerous pregnancies. Although this was a mixed bag for Sanger, since she was not really pro-condom as a birth control option (and her area of concern was not really disease prevention), the ruling turned the condom into a legitimate device and opened up the doors to new business opportunities. And it once and for all killed the Comstock Act.

> ## SANGER'S PAMPHLETS
> The birth control booklet that got Sanger's husband arrested was called What Every Girl Should Know. When a box of them was returned to her after being confiscated by federal agents, she noticed that under the title of the booklets, a witty agent had written "NOTHING, by order of the Post Office Department." This was, after all, an America where buying a single condom made the buyer and the seller criminals in thirty states; where priests told women who used black-market diaphragms that they would be haunted by the faces of their unborn children; and where some women like Sanger's devoutly Catholic mother, who got pregnant eighteen times and had eleven children and seven miscarriages, died an early death from the ravages of so many births.

Just before the war ended in 1918, American condoms were sold publicly for the first time in forty-five years. The Comstock Act, along with Comstock himself, was dead—but it was too late for all those soldiers who had not been able to access practical prophylaxis.

And although the British had never tried to ban sales, and wiser heads had helped provide the British military with necessary prophylaxis, throughout the twenties, there would still be those who tried their best to make the condom a dirty little secret.

> ## THE CASE OF BALTIMORE
> In a study on condom use, it was found that just prior to World War I in Baltimore alone, about three million were sold per year. By 1920 that number had more than doubled.

ELEVEN

nookie in the struggle buggy

ALL THAT JAZZ AND THE AGE OF ADVERTISING

*A*fter the sexually confused Victorian era and the devastating war were over, it was time to "live again." Many young people took advantage of the rapidly changing social norms to break with old conventions. Provocative terms like *spooning, petting, "it" girl, vamps, flappers,* and *gaiety girls* became part of contemporary language. Young women rebelled against old-fashioned mores by raising their hem lengths, cutting their hair into "bobs," and "picking up" men. Reflecting on the changes in courting in the United States, in 1927 Emily Post's book of etiquette talked about the "Vanishing Chaperon," or as young men called them, "fire extinguishers." Young couples were no longer accompanied on their *dates*, yet another new love word.

In the United Kingdom, the *Bright Young Things* were slammed by the conservative press, but enjoyed a sexual freedom, first experienced by those who had served as nurses and ambulance drivers during World War I, unbeknownst to their mothers and grandmothers. The term the "Jazz Age" became a synonym for sex.

For Americans, the 1920s was the first era in which most people lived in cities, a complete reversal from just a few decades before when the majority still lived on farms. Life expectancy for the country's population of 106 million was the highest in history—men could expect to live to fifty-three and women, fifty-four, ten years more than the previous generation. The military had only 343,000 men, down from well over a million in 1919. The average man made a whopping $1,236 a year, and illiteracy was at its lowest level ever—94 percent of Americans could read and write. Wall Street came into its own, and Madison Avenue was born. *And*, the prohibition against producing and drinking alcohol combined with rampant corruption in many police departments made the twenties an era when gangland crime and mob warfare went unchecked.

For the English, things were not quite so rosy, as industry never recovered from the effects of war and the labor movement had really begun in earnest, putting added pressures on the economy and on the country's social structure. For all that, however, the children of the aristocracy and the middle classes were having a jolly good time, sipping cocktails, speaking dribble, and generally enjoying doing little of consequence.

THE MODEL-T AND NO MORE FIRE EXTINGUISHERS

SEXY STATISTICS
With the birth of sociological studies and statistics, for the first time in American history, there were reliable figures about what Americans were doing "behind closed doors." In a 1925 sex study it was found that thirty out of fifty women under the age of forty had had premarital sex. By the 1930s, it was over 50 percent, only slightly less than the war years.

According to a report by American sociologists (a new profession that arose out of progressivism) Robert and Helen Lynd, by the early twenties young people were in a world of their own, no longer bound by the mores and morals of their parents and grandparents; the Lynds' study showed that 50 percent of young adults living in urban areas identified themselves as sexually active. This was due to the general loosening of morals . . . *and the car.*

In the United States, Henry Ford's mass-produced automobiles made it possible for even working-class Americans to afford to buy one. But Ford's little black car was dubbed a "house of prostitution on wheels" by worried mothers and fathers, and admonitions not to "park" were heard across America. Worries or not, *nookie in the struggle buggy*—sex in the backseat of the car—was here to stay.

"RED TIPS FOR HOT LIPS"

Modern marketing techniques became the key to good sales in the 1920s. Although condom sales had been incredible during the war, by 1920 Europeans were manufacturing their own again, and American manufacturers floundered in the first few years of the new decade. Looking for ways to beef up the market, they borrowed new marketing ideas being used to sell other products.

Catchy names and slick packaging were especially important for the condom industry because prophylactics could only be labeled and sold legally as disease preventatives. Influenced by the way cigarettes (now premade instead of hand rolled, handsomely packaged, and designed with colored paper ends inspired by the British brand Red Tips) were being marketed, condom manufacturers began to package their wares in slick little "cigarette" cases, three to a package, subtle and perfectly sized for a man's pocket. Easy access was important when the petting party went "all the way."

Packaging helped the producers work around legal restrictions on how their products were labeled. They

> ## CIVILIZED VOODOO
> The new morals of the Jazz Age had plenty of detractors. The Ladies' Home Journal *described the birth of jazz as "originally . . . the accompaniment of the voodoo dancer, stimulating the half-crazed barbarian to the vilest deeds," while the new music showed a "blatant disregard of even the elementary rules of civilization" because jazz was strictly "whorehouse music" and "music in the nude." The author does not disclose how he came up with this jazz provenance.*

> ## RAMSES FOR WOMEN
> Schmid had also diversified by the early twenties and was manufacturing diaphragms. Capitalizing on his popular Ramses prophylactic and the newly established importance of brand names, he also called his women's product "Ramses," though the name recognition did not increase its sales.

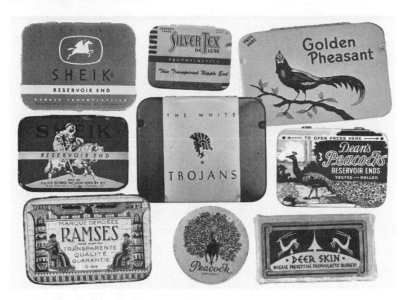

Condom tins from the 1910s to the 1930s

made their brand names stand out and the images on the packages sexy. Although benign and downright dull terms like "liquid latex" or "liquid latex prophylactic rubbers" were used to describe the contents of the package, the brand names often reflected gently erotic themes; Julius Schmid's Sheiks exploited the popularity of Rudolph Valentino, who was referred to as "the Sheik," a twenties euphemism for the sensuous man. Schmid also produced the Ramses brand, with its picture of an Egyptian king on the front inferring that the man who wore one was as sexually powerful as an Egyptian pharoah. His others were not quite as colorful, but still had suggestive names like Fourex, Paradise, and Velveto. Other brands like Parisians were identifying themselves with the new postwar language that found all things French risqué—and it was not a far leap from the still-common French letters.

The Merry Widows were more popular for their unique packaging and message than for their quality. The widows came in a little round gold can with three condoms tucked neatly in their waxy little wrappings, each with

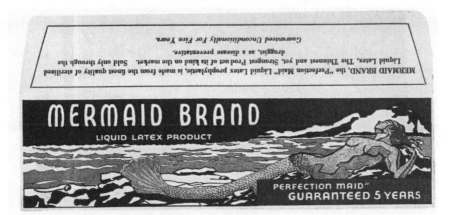

The sexy mermaid

its own name—Agnes, Mabel, and Beckie. The sophisticated marketing implied that sexually savvy women loved this brand best.

For their purely sensual message, however, Mermaids had to win the prize. This condom package was labeled "Perfection maid," and was decorated with a very seductive sea maiden, leaning back in an erotic pose, lounging topless on a rock. Hardly subtle, but very effective.

Britons continued to enjoy the only British-made protection, the Durex, but most of theirs were unremarkably packaged preservatifs, imported once again from Germany.

❋❋❋

There were other packaging innovations in the twenties, but they were of a more practical nature; in the 1920s, Dupont engineers developed a new material they called cellophane and some of the top condom manufacturers used it to improve the shelf life of their product. Better yet, a new and improved Trojan made from a revolutionary rubber product called latex made its debut in 1920.

Condom sales skyrocketed in the Jazz Age.

LATEX AND DREADNOUGHTS

In the 1910s, Julius Schmid had introduced the first major rubber innovation since Goodyear had figured out the vulcanization process. He pioneered the cement-dipping method.

Dipping required the same glass molds that had been used by the more refined gut makers for centuries, but they were now dunked in large vats of a liquid rubber solution rather than wrapped with strips of premade rubber or gutta percha. As revolutionary as the process was, however, Schmid's new technique had some unfortunate side effects.

Because gasoline or benzene had to be added to the imported sap to make it truly liquid, the problem with cement dipping was that the improved rubber product was highly flammable in its liquid state. Since there was always the threat of fire from a variety of sources at the production plants—even the spark from a piece of electrical equipment could ignite a vat of rubber—the big players, all of whom had had to contend with fires and the ensuing loss of revenue and equipment, began to take out insurance on their factories. Because of the high risk, the premiums were steep, but for the larger manufacturers it was cheaper than the cost of a fire. Then along came latex.

Latex helped cut the cost of insurance by eliminating the flammability problem. It required only water to suspend the liquid sap and simplified the production process; the penis molds were dipped into the latex, and then cured in warm water . . . no more rubbing, trimming, but most important, no more chemicals. The final product looked nicer, could be stored for up to five years (the old rubbers, in spite of what the advertising claimed, had a shelf life of only three months), and was stronger yet a lot thinner, making it much more sensitive.

Oddly, latex represents yet another of the funny little coincidences in the life of the humble condom. Throughout the 1920s, some of the finest scientists in the United States worked on the "latex project," hoping to help medicine by making much-improved surgical gloves, but inadvertently improved another little device and earned it a place in the history of serious science.

Although by the beginning of the twenties Americans were buying millions of latex condoms per day, the more refined latex *American letter* did not arrive on European shores until the end of the decade. The first latex sheath to appear on the English market in 1929 was an export, manufactured by the US Youngs Rubber Corporation; although it was essentially a Trojan, the British labeled it under the not-very-subtle name Dreadnought instead. By 1932, the London Rubber Company, which had previously been a wholesale business importing German preser-vatifs, began to produce its own latex rubbers in competition with the American market.

> ## WHAT'S IN A NAME?
> *It may have been possible that Merle Youngs was a fan of Shakespeare, influencing his decision to name history's most famous brand of condom. In Troilus and Cressida, the unfaithful "quondam wife" of Greek Menelaus— Helen—prefers Trojan men to Greeks.*

AUTOMATED PROPHYLACTICS

Throughout the twenties, latex and cement-dipped condoms were still handmade, requiring the big producers to employ a lot of semiskilled workers, but with the advancement of the assembly line, the brainchild of a new breed called the "engineer" and embraced by industrialists like Ford, even the condom industry went high tech.

The first real condom assembly line involved a series of hands-on activities, including the specialized job of rolling the open end of each rubber in order to have a smooth, finished edge. But that cumbersome chore was eliminated when in 1926, Fred Killian of Akron, Ohio, invented and patented the first automatic condom "ring" machine. Killian's new invention ended the need for workers to perform the rolling function, and sped up the process considerably.

By 1930, Killian, manufacturer of the Perma-Tex and Silver-Tex condom brands, had improved upon his design and produced a complete assembly line (originally intended only for his own plant). The new system required almost no hands-on involvement during the production process. Although there are no surviving photographs of the line, the patent describes an amazing conveyor belt that automatically dipped four thousand glass "forms" or "bottles" into ivory-colored latex, one dip per second. The mold holders were designed to move back and forth, from side to side, in order to prevent the tip of the condom from forming a "nipple" shape or unattractive lumps and bumps that would make them less than aesthetic. Cylinder-shaped brushes rolled the top of the condom to finish the open edge, and then blasts of hot air and a dip in hot water vulcanized—finished off and sealed—it.

An assembly line attendant sprinkled talcum powder on every one of the finished products, which helped dry the rubber and make them smooth, and then they were removed by another set of brushes that scraped each off of its original mold. The roughly rolled product was conveyed down to the only people who actually touched them—until after being sold. Women workers stretched out each condom—they tended to bunch up when removed from the mold—making sure each was straight because newly formed latex tended to "glue" together if it was not straightened out right after processing. Then the molds went through a cleansing hot water bath to remove any contaminants before beginning the whole process again.

This new, twenty-four-hour-a-day production method meant a much better product at a much lower production price, and thousands of condoms a day could be produced without fear of fire or human error. Killian's invention was so successful, after patenting it, he went public and charged a whopping $20,000 (as much as $2 million today) per conveyor system. Sales were limited, but the big boys snapped them up; others took advantage of Killian's leasing program, the terms of which included that the leasee had to pay Fred Killian a percentage of the total sales resultant from production. The high cost of purchase meant that in just one decade, none of the

CONDOM CARPAL TUNNEL SYNDROME

Although the new technology of the 1920s had eliminated of a lot of the tedious jobs like dipping, through the end of the 1950s women (who were the majority of the workers in big condom factories) often complained of the aches and pains they suffered. At Schmid's New Jersey factory, which employed thousands of women to do the quality checks and other repetitive jobs, workers complained of what today we know as carpal tunnel syndrome.

remaining small condom manufacturers could hold their own in the marketplace, making this once-small entrepreneur-friendly business one of the top moneymakers in American industry; men like Schmid and Youngs found themselves squarely in the middle of Wall Street, two of only fifteen major manufacturers left by 1925.

THE COIN-OPERATED CONDOM

The Germans were back in production by the early twenties, once again dominating the European condom market and kicking the American condom back across the Atlantic. One German manufacturer sold more than twenty-four million a year throughout the decade. They had also, along with the Dutch, pioneered the slot, or vending, machine in the late 1910s. By the 1920s, condom vending machines were all over the United States, Germany, the Netherlands, and England. The highly public sales venue and the easy consumer access was symbolic of the incredible impact industrialization had had on Western nations, and how universally accepted the condom had become.

CAVEAT EMPTOR!

Condom magnate Julius Schmid, the man who had arrived on American shores with only the shirt on his back, sold twenty million latex condoms in one year alone in the 1920s, making him second only to Youngs in production. But just because letters had gone high tech, high profile, and big business, it did not mean that all was well in condomland, at least not ethically speaking.

THE "TIE MAN"

Men carrying small suitcases, a travel innovation of the 1890s, were seen in many urban areas throughout the 1920s. Door-to-door peddlers, these men sold just about anything that was small and portable, and were often hassled by the local constabulary as "disturbers of the peace." Finding a special niche in the crowded office ghettos of large towns and cities, the one breed of peddlers, or the "tie man," was somewhat unique: his case contained a dozen or so cheap ties on top, but had a false bottom from which he sold condoms. Buying from the tie man became a Jazz Age euphemism for purchasing condoms.

Although the tremendous boon in manufacturing improvements meant better condoms, the testing process was still necessary to assure safety and effectiveness. To be sure of their products, and to be able to guarantee consistent quality, manufacturers like Schmid employed dozens of women whose sole job it was to check each rubber for holes, dirt, and other contaminants. The process added to the production and sales price, but made his brands very popular with choosy consumers. In spite of this quality testing, though, in the big, bad world of condom commerce it was still buyer beware.

The first generation of Trojans went into production in 1916. But after the war, Youngs (who had started out in the business under the name Youngs and Fey) had struggled because of the drop in exports to Europe. The new Trojans had put US Youngs Rubber Corporation back on the map because of their comfort and reliability; latex and testing made that possible. The problem was the rejects.

Once a Trojan had been found to be defective, it was discarded into a cardboard box underneath the quality-control conveyor belts, but contrary to ethical business practice, these defectives were not thrown away at the end of the day. Instead, they were quietly sealed up and put in the warehouse, and surreptitiously sold later as seconds to less-than-reputable "jobbers" who were always able to find outlets for really cheap rubbers: barbershops, gas stations, shoe shine boys, and bartenders at speakeasies all bought and sold them.

As big a player in the business as Youngs was (he even had a Standard & Poor's rating), he was too cheap (and to be fair, he had struggled to keep his business afloat after the war) to throw away the rejects, and he made a tidy profit from selling his defects to wholesalers. Youngs's accountants called his seconds "different grades" in their account books, but this side business actually added a healthy addition to his bottom line. Although he himself never suffered any negative consequences for his dishonesty, Youngs's lack of ethics did have its price.

WHAT'S IN A NAME?

Manufacturers moved beyond just trendy packaging when they again took their cue from other industries and began to apply for trademarks for their products. They also moved away from the small, surreptitious advertisements of the old days, taking out whole-page ads in major papers around the country, selling their condoms as *disease preventers*.

It was Merle Youngs who took marketing well beyond vending machines, packaging, and newspapers, though. He decided that he could capture a serious market share for his best products, selling them through only one venue. His reasoning was that since his products could only be labeled as disease preventatives, it made sense to sell his Trojans through pharmacies. After all, pharmacists were trusted corner retailers who were always dispensing advice about their products. Youngs saw the chance to take advantage of a free sales force. He sold pharmacists on the idea by emphasizing the fact that Trojans were the most reliable on the market; by pushing them over other brands, the pharmacists were differentiating themselves as true professionals who offered only the finest (disease) protection. The high price they fetched did not hurt their feelings, either.

Publicly, he couched this sales strategy not as a moneymaking scheme, but as one based on Youngs's deeply held belief that he must protect his customers from harm. He wanted American men to feel safe when they used his brand. But the reality was that by narrowing his outlets to pharmacists only, Youngs could sell Trojans at a premium price—and he was capitalizing on the fact that many people work off the premise that the more expensive a product is, the better quality it must be. Youngs's Trojans brand sold for $1.50 a dozen (at least $15 today, adjusting for inflation), while the lesser brands (like Merry Widows) cost less than a third of that. The lesser prophylactics were sold at a variety of outlets, but they did not have the snob appeal Trojans had cultivated throughout the twenties.

Pharmacists were an important part of the success of the Trojans brand and Youngs got his wish. Pharmacies set a high-profit margin for the premium product, which "paid the rent" for pharmacists across the country . . . and Youngs got his free sales force.

The two distinct marketing techniques Youngs employed worked in tandem; by pushing his Trojans through a "health" retailer and by supplying imperfect prophylactics to jobbers who sold them to anyone who was buying, he exploited both ends of the market. Experience with bad condoms might have left some men—and women—figuring that higher-priced sheaths were worth the cost. He also conveniently blamed his competitors—some who sold off their "seconds" and others who never bothered to test their products—for any bad image problems, never admitting to his own contribution to that poor reputation.

The producer of Trojans also inadvertently helped to make the big manufacturers even bigger when a former customer (who had purchased resale seconds from Youngs) was angered after being told that Youngs would no longer sell to him, possibly due to a personal argument between the two. The angry jobber decided to get back at Youngs by borrowing the Trojan label, stamping it on rejects he purchased from another manufacturer, and selling his goods as the genuine article. Reminiscent of the battling Mrs. P's of eighteenth-century England, an advertising war ensued, and Youngs, who had received a trademark patent for Trojans a few years before, sued the jobber for trademark infringement, claiming he had the exclusive right to use the Trojans label.

The Trojan War had begun.

THE MORE THINGS CHANGE, THE MORE THEY STAY THE SAME

It was a test case, since condoms had pretty much been confined to criminal court cases involving activists like Margaret Sanger and the small-time dealers of the nineteenth century who were unlucky enough to get caught by Anthony Comstock.

The first judge to hear the Youngs's trademark infringement case was someone out of the bad old days of condom controversy. He flatly stated that it was not a legitimate legal case and dismissed it, claiming that the suit was contrary to "public morals and an aid to and an encourager of lewdness and lechery," thereby "sufficiently reprehensible to outside the field of equitable protection." But Youngs was a tough cookie and a survivor of years of this kind of legal prejudice. He took the case back to court in 1930, and a judge on the US Court of Appeals for the Second Circuit saw it differently.

Reflecting the changing face of American society and at the same time harking back to the hypocrisy that is the history of the condom, the US Court of Appeals sided with Youngs, stating that Trojans was a legal trademark for a "legitimate disease preventative." Happy news for Youngs and his sales force. Now, all the big manufacturers could rest easy about spending large amounts on advertising their wares without fear of trademark infringement or shaky legal standing of their prod-

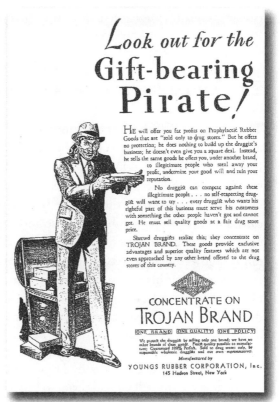

The "Trojan Wars" begin

ucts because they were "contrary to public morals." But the judge's view that Mr. Youngs's decision to market only through legitimate pharmacists, keeping prophylactics in a medicinal light rather than as a dirty little sex aid, just perpetuated the lie and illustrated the same old illogic that has dogged the condom for centuries. The judge made it clear that condoms sold through a pharmacy were a "promoter of health," while the lesser brands (especially those produced by smaller makers and not marketed through pharmacies) were obviously used during illicit sexual encounters because they were being sold through illegitimate nonmedical outlets.

Unperturbed by legal hypocrisy, and as brand-name recognition became more and more important to their sales, by 1930 the big manufacturers had all applied for patents. Just a few years before men had bought rubbers, sheaths, or letters; now they had to decide between Trojans, Ramses, Sheiks, and Mermaids.

TWO AND SIXPENCE AND A BLOB OF SEALING WAX

There were no British court cases fought over condom trademarks nor were manufacturers restricted to selling their prophylactics only as disease preventatives. Durexes and Dreadnoughts were openly advertised as birth control. This enlightened approach to regulation and marketing make it all the more curious then that, though the British had embraced, before Americans, a more open policy about the use and sales of sheaths, when it came to condom sales, many British chemists behaved as if they were selling—reluctantly—government secrets instead of rubbers.

Recollecting his experiences as an apprentice in the 1920s, a British chemist laughed as he described the awkwardness of customers because of the disapproval of his fellow chemists when there was a request for a "package":

> The awkwardness . . . arose from the ritual involved in supplying them. A customer who did not already know first had the embarrassment of finding out if the shop sold them. When a solitary man came in, asked loudly for a tube of toothpaste and then lingered anxiously while the girl assistants discreetly disappeared, you knew what he really wanted. The matter did not end there. When at last he eventually found the courage to lean over the counter and whisper, his requirement still had to be met.
>
> The articles were kept, no less securely than the dangerous drugs, locked in the safe next to the cash box. The junior apprentice was not really supposed to know, so the forbidden word was passed quietly along the line to one of the pharmacists. Then, with eyes averted and sometimes a slight reddening of the cheeks, he would grope blindly on the top shelf of the safe, hastily wrap something in plain white paper, apply a blob of sealing wax, and hand it to the customer himself, saying "take two and sixpence, Charles." It was all very awkward.

Another young apprentice also described his experiences selling French letters as a very hush-hush affair:

Oh, very, very, under the counter. Only the pharmacists sold them. I wasn't allowed to sell them. In fact, I was not shown where the Durex was kept. They were in a drawer. I discovered that because I could go anywhere I liked, but I discovered those on my own. That was rather like the whole conception of birth and everything between parents and their children. You sort of grew into the knowledge, and my apprentice master very much followed that. And no one sold Durex to the customers except the pharmacist. The customers would come in and say "may I see Mr. Elder, please?" or "may I see the pharmacist?" Of course, every member of the staff knew exactly what they wanted, but that was the attitude. Very much under the counter.

This odd prejudice was so pervasive that the United Kingdom's largest and most famous (and still in business today) pharmacy chain, Boots, decided in the twenties to adopt a policy against selling condoms, claiming the new rule was to protect its staff from having to deal with any "awkwardness." The Boots staff, on the other hand, was not quite so positive about this odd policy. A longtime employee recalled her experiences as a clerk:

> Boots only sold contraceptive pessaries. There were not many requests for the *sheath*—most people seemed to know that Boots didn't sell them. But occasionally we would get requests. They would come in and say "packet of Durex please." You would say "sorry, we don't sell them." They would ask "why don't you sell them?" And we would say that the company doesn't allow us to sell them. "Why's that then?" "Because they feel it's embarrassing for the staff." "Well, it's a darn sight more embarrassing for the staff when I come in here and ask for them and they have to explain to me why they can't sell them."
>
> That was the sort of reaction you would get. So it was a lot more embarrassing for the staff. At least (if you had them) you could slip them into a bag and pass them over the counter; it was a lot less fuss than trying to explain why you couldn't sell them in the first place.

Boots did not reverse that policy until the 1960s.

And it was not until well after World War II that the leading agency that had been influential in convincing some independent pharmacies not to sell sheaths began to reverse its anticondom stance. The English Pharmaceutical Society began by telling its members, "There should be no exhibition of contraceptive in a pharmacy, or any reference by way of advertisement, notice, show-card or otherwise that they are sold there, other than a notice approved by the Council bearing the world 'Family Planning Requisites.'" All very droll.

Unperturbed by this silliness, throughout the teens and twenties, most Englishmen ordered out of catalogs or went to specialty stores, a vending machine, the barber, or a "rubber goods" store for their "little something for the weekend."

PROPHYLACTIC POPULARITY

Throughout the twenties, condom sales in countries around the world doubled. In the United States, the condom business had joined the rest of the big boys on Wall Street—its advanced production techniques, assembly lines, legal backing, and a booming market influenced by the continued lightening up of sexual mores all contributed to making condom production an incredibly profitable industry. And like all trends, its public acceptance meant that it even showed up in popular fiction. In his best-selling book *Manhattan Transfer*, John Dos Passos documented another common twenties euphemism for the condom by having one of his leading characters worried about his "propho."

In spite of the public acceptance of the propho and its availability through legitimate retail, many American men, like their British counterparts, still bought their supplies from street salesmen, barbers, bartenders, at the gas station, corner delicatessen, candy store, from shoeshine boys, tobacconists, restaurant waitstaff, baggers at the grocers, bellhops, and even at the tailors! Those still living in the more rural areas could order their supplies through the mail from catalogs. Sears and Roebuck sold a variety of sheaths, along with other devices that were obviously intended for birth control. It seemed everyone was in on the condom action, taking advantage of the fact that Americans were more sexually active than ever before.

A FREUDIAN "SLIP"—THE PROS AND CONS

Although he had written about his dislike of the condom as early as 1895, by the 1920s Austrian psychoanalyst Sigmund Freud was more vociferous in his comments about the little device; he maintained that the sheath cut down on sexual pleasure and that it "hurt the fine susceptibilities of both partners." He was critical of all types of birth control—claiming he was concerned that no method was foolproof—but he reserved his greatest contempt for the condom. Freudian scholars postulate that his extreme dislike of the sheath was because of its disruptive quality and, most probably, his love-hate relationship with sex all the way around.

Other high-visibility Jazz Age opponents of the condom included a well-known woman doctor, Dorothy Bocker. Bocker worked in Margaret Sanger's New York birth control clinic in the early twenties, where she came to dislike the condom on the same grounds earlier birth control advocates had stated—it took control away from women, it was not regulated by doctors, "breakage" could be a problem, and it was awkward to use, possibly discouraging regular use.

In Great Britain, there was some debate over whether condom use could be considered moral. The Church of England's 1920 Lambeth conference condemned the use of "unnatural means of conception avoidance." It warned against the physical, moral, and religious dangers of using any kind of contraceptive. The bishop of London, a prominent member of numerous "public morality councils" who was deemed by one of his detractors a "still-single fuss budget," tried to stop all pharmacists from selling condoms—without success.

Bishop Arthur Winnington-Ingram fought against anything he felt added to the seedier side of London life, but he had an especially virulent dislike of condoms, constantly complaining about the huge number of them discarded in alleyways and parks all over the city. The problem was most acute after weekends and holidays when legions of dustmen were sent out to collect and dispose of them. Railing against the used sheaths, the bishop said, "I would like to make a bonfire of them and dance round it." Talk about Freudian.

The British medical journal the *Lancet* also showed distain for the condom, dismissing it as a "distasteful subject . . . impotent to deal with any certainty with the virile spermatozoon." Others in the medical field warned of the horror a young wife would experience if she were exposed to something as shocking as her new husband donning his letter. And the old chestnut about using a condom was tantamount to masturbation, or "masturbation à deux," had not gone away either.

Other detractors did not care about the rights and wrongs of its use; they simply demanded the closure of "rubber shops" because they represented a moral danger on "visual grounds."

IGNORE THE OBSCURANTISTS!

Arguments for condom use during the 1920s far outweighed the arguments against it. When author H. G. Wells, who sat on the board of the National Birth Control Council with Marie Stopes, heard people argue against birth control, he informed them that all Britons had the right, and the need, to be informed about sex, contraception, and the devices necessary to protect themselves. Wells argued that birth control protected women: "I think that a married woman who knows nothing about birth control is little better than a serf, a mere helpless breeding animal, and when I find an obscurantist Roman Catholic sitting in the light at the Ministry of Health, I think myself entitled to make a noise about it."

Wells was joined by the more liberal Church of England clergymen who outnumbered the conservatives, calling for "a more definite statement as to how Christian men and women may live their married lives in harmony with Church principles and Bible teaching, and yet not bring into the world children for whom they can see no prospect of making reasonable provision." The bishop of Birmingham was more blunt about it: "We must have a recognition of the legitimacy of birth-control."

The old Malthusian concerns over birthrate among the poor also remained a concern for some. Educated laymen and doctors alike spoke out for sex education for the poor as an important health measure and called for "sheath use" to prevent too many pregnancies.

Elsewhere in Europe, pro and con debates raged, especially in France. Concerned about the depopulation caused by the terrible death toll of World War I, French conservatives called on their fellow parliamentarians to make birth control illegal because of the "most urgent need to increase [French] natality." Indicative of how the pendulum had swung in that nation, the few who argued that such a draconian act would simply lead to underground black marketing of devices were booed. When Communist Andre Berthon asked, "Are you going to condemn pharmacists who sell . . . let's speak plainly . . . condoms?" he barely made it out of the chamber without bodily injury.

The sole pro-condom voice in the Republican Party was a gynecologist and member of the Extra Parliamentary Commission on Depopulation. His objection to turning around centuries-old acceptance and use of a variety of birth control and disease preventative measures was based on his medical experiences; he was convinced that women who did not have access to implements would end up using "penholders" to solve the problem of unwanted pregnancy. A precautionary note for the decades to come.

VIRILE PROTECTORS

The loosening of sexual mores in the Jazz Age is actually credited with helping to contribute to a drop in the number of prostitutes and brothels in the United States and Europe, which paralleled a drop in the number of venereal diseases reported throughout the twenties. In spite of the statistics, which they may or may not have been aware of, military leaders were still concerned about sexually transmitted diseases and the threat they posed for sailors and soldiers.

The British and other European militaries continued to supply their members with prophylactics. Even the ultraconservative, anti–birth control, future Fascist leader of Spain, General Francisco Franco, required his army cadets be supplied with German-made condoms when they went out

at night. He did spot checks as the young men left for an evening of enjoyment, and was known to extract severe punishments if anyone was caught
not carrying at least one letter. But it was not until 1927 that the American
army and navy finally saw the light in regard to prevention rather than cure.
Senior medical officers promoted the use of educational programs, along
with making *protectors* easily available.

In order to gain acceptance for making condoms a part of any sailor's or
soldier's kit, the military turned the old abstinence and purity campaign
around and made virility the center of their argument—an army or navy
made up of emasculated men, with no sex drive, was unthinkable! The
"boys will be boys" approach worked. Helped by the general lessening of old
traditions and prudish Victorian sexual taboos, prophylactics were easily
found at any military site around the world, and were standard issue to all
American military members by 1931. The lessons from the Great War had
finally been learned.

TWELVE

brother, can you spare a dime . . . for a rubber?

THE GREAT DEPRESSION

hen the American stock market crashed and burned in 1929, the halcyon days of the Jazz Age were over, and the lighthearted belief that the good times would never end were replaced with the worst economic depression in history. Millions of American men were out of work, with many of the unemployed living the hobo's life or packing everything they could into the old Model-T to search for a better place.

Although few Americans were spared the pain, there were some bright spots in an otherwise bleak time. In 1930, to the delight of many little girls, Nancy Drew began to solve her mysteries; the *Better Homes and Gardens Cookbook* went on sale, one day to join the short list of the best-selling books in history; games like Monopoly were created to help wile away long hours at home; Castle Burgers was the first fast-food chain, serving an affordable little five-cent burger; and two out of every five homes in America had a radio ushering in the Golden Age of Broadcast, with celebrities like Bing Crosby, Guy Lombardo, and Rudy Vallee dominating the airwaves. Because few could afford to enjoy the more lavish entertainments so popular in the twenties, Depression-era Hollywood, helped by the arrival of color film, prospered. Millions of Americans scraped up a quarter every week to sit in a theater and lose themselves in the films of Clark Gable, Judy Garland, and Katharine Hepburn.

And, there was no Black Friday for the condom.

There were a number of factors that helped the Depression-era condom business flourish—some legal, most financial. Although the law was always behind the times, several US Federal Court of Appeals cases finally repealed the last of the federal "Comstock leftovers." For the first time, doctors were free to prescribe preventatives for any reason they deemed fit. Although very few men or women consulted doctors when it came to contraception, the decision prompted the old-fashioned American Medical Association to finally withdraw its objections to the condom as birth control. This paved the way in 1938 for more than three hundred *legal* birth control clinics to open across the country, supplying poor women with condoms, diaphragms, and general medical help and advice. Longtime followers of Margaret Sanger were at once disgusted that it had taken so many years for it to happen and delighted that finally poor women had free and legal birth control options.

An even more important legal decision assisted the industry in a big way: a federal court ended the Comstock-era ban on the advertising of birth control information, making it legal to advertise and ship prophylactics. Although mail-order catalogs had been doing a land-office business for years, this made it much easier for the well-respected catalogs like Sears and Roebuck to now *boldly* market their brands, which not only made the products more visible but also helped to continue educating the public about condom use.

Also at the federal level, in spite of cuts in budgets that meant less money to supply troops with their kits, the American army and navy continued with their policy of quietly adding pros to the standard provisions given to soldiers and sailors. Although military leaders claimed this was just a continuation of the 1918 decision to provide prophylaxis for disease protection, since that time, the navy had actually handed out printed materials informing its men that their kits were also handy for birth control. Married military men used as many pros as unmarried. When he ran out of the free-bies and had to buy his own, the average military member was paying ten cents (roughly a dollar today) for a box of three at his local exchange. A study from the early thirties conducted by the surgeon general on the pur-chase of condoms at army bases indicated that even when soldiers had to pay for their own, they did so willingly, buying an average of ten per soldier, per year. The provision of the kits along with easy access on base coincided with a steep decline in venereal diseases reported by the military.

"I CAN'T GIVE YOU ANYTHING BUT LOVE, BABY" . . . WORDS OF ROMANCE IN TIMES OF TROUBLE

The sexy slang of the Depression is deeply reflective of the feelings of helplessness of the times. They also illustrate the ever-increasing public acceptance of more open sexual behaviors. On the make, whanger, and impotence were used by men and women, and were featured in some of the most important fiction of the era. The Grapes of Wrath featured screw, pecker, trigger, dong, and lay, as well as references to contraception.

Although dropping the legal barriers to advertising condoms as birth con-trol and the continued push for their use by the military certainly helped support the booming industry, the real reason for the amazing sales during the Depression was that fewer and fewer Americans felt they could afford to have children. No matter how broke couples were, they could find a few cents to prevent pregnancy. Condoms were cheaper than children.

The need to have fewer, or no, children conflicted with the fact that with such high unemployment, adults had a lot more time on their hands. During the sexy twenties, the taboo that made having sex during the day a no-no had dropped; there were plenty of people using their little devices for afternoon delights.

Because of the social and financial pressures so many people were under, fewer and fewer couples felt they could even afford to marry, and the marriage rate dropped like a stone. By 1935 there were fewer marriages being performed than at any other time in American history, which meant an even greater need to prevent unwanted pregnancies; it is perhaps a cruel irony that in a time of such financial ruin, during every year of the Depression, people spent more than thirty-three million dollars on condoms.

BUST AND BOOM

During the Depression, American manufacturers churned out more than 1.5 million condoms a day. The word *condom*, however, remained something men muttered only among themselves, most preferring the popular euphemisms of the day: *safety, rubber, overcoat, raincoat, French cap, French letter, nodder, protection, pro, rubber Johnny,* and *propho*. Women favored just *widow*.

Like their American counterparts, European manufacturers continued to enjoy great sales, and both American and British men bought their supplies from the same sources as before: coin-operated machines, local barbershops, and gas (petrol) stations. In spite of the worldwide impact of the

> **MALCOLM X**
> Before his activist career, Malcolm X survived the Depression by selling condoms to patrons at local Boston dance halls.

crash, European and English condom producers did very well for themselves. In 1932 the London Rubber Company, which had only been a wholesaler for German sheaths prior to this time, began to produce its own latex *nodders* (a British euphemism). The company became Britain's largest manufacturer, producing about two million per year.

NOT QUITE FULLER BRUSH, BUT . . .

The unique marketplace, along with the creativity that is often the result of desperation, may help explain the rise of a new kind of entrepreneur—the prophylactic door-to-door salesman. Taking their cue from generations of peddlers, a profession that was revived in the Jazz Age with the creation of the Fuller Brush Man, this sales force was made of up of men who traveled as far as necessary to sell their (not very good) "rubber goods." Many women across America had the unusual experience of opening their doors to be greeted with a cheery "Good morning, madam, have you a moment to view my excellent *preventatives*?" Although the peddlers did not make a lot of money or challenge the profits of the retail sales outlets, these independents did have their own small market share, apparently acceptable in the topsy-turvy world of the Great Depression.

Even though sales venues altered little—with the exception of door-to-door sales—the industry itself went through major changes in the thirties, leaving behind most of its ancient roots, and solidifying its new role as a big player in the world of commerce. At the same time, Casanova's old complaint had not gone away.

THE NUMBERS GAME

The high startup costs, especially the invention of Killian's condom conveyor in 1930, meant that by the midthirties only a handful of major manufacturers remained in the market, a continuation of the consolidation that had begun in the 1920s. Youngs Rubber Company, Julius Schmid, Inc., Louis Shunk, and the Dean Rubber Manufacturing Company were the biggest players, followed by lesser (but profitable) companies like Atlanta's Olympia Laboratory. Youngs's now-famous latex Trojans brand was one of the most popular because of its reliability, but it was too expensive for many.

Ever savvy when it came to understanding the market niche for his sheaths, Schmid had stuck with the old cement rubber technique. Although it meant his factories had a greater incidence of fire, Julius felt it worth the risk; by using the old method of production, he could legitimately label his rubbers as longer lasting—reusable—and they did stand up to the kinds of lubricants (animal fats and Vaseline) still used after more than fifty years. Choosy consumers had long since abandoned this practice, but during the Depression low price and reusability were appealing for those who needed to economize.

Production figures differ from company to company, but the general cost of doing business breaks down to approximately $2.20 per gross. The rubber and chemicals accounted for about 20¢ per gross; 40¢ went to overhead; $1.30 to the sales force; and anywhere from nothing to 25¢ per gross was spent on testing. Everything else was for miscellaneous procedures, depending on the quality and manufacturing process. The excessively high marketing cost versus a relatively low cost of production was driven by the fact that the condom market was no longer a mostly urban one; Americans everywhere wanted them and that meant a widespread sales force and higher shipping costs.

Bulk condoms could be purchased by distributors, some for as little as 50¢ a gross. They were the "generics" packaged under a variety of names, most lost to history. Others went for anywhere from $1.50 to almost $11 per gross. The higher-end condoms were produced by the top three manufacturers and sold under their labels. Those sold at gas stations, and from vending machines, barbers, bartenders, corner food shops, pool halls, and bellhops were of poor quality, and went for as little as three for 75¢, but that was still a high profit considering the barber would have paid only $6 for a gross. In spite of the lower quality, men found it more convenient to get their

> ## THE FRENCH SKIN, ALIVE AND WELL
> *In spite of the intense poverty suffered by so many, there remained a mostly underground market for fine imported French skins. These were purchased by those men who went unscathed—and even profited from—the crash. Although they were not a significant percentage of the market, skins remained popular with that exclusive group. The imported French letter was still produced from fine animal intestine and smuggled in to avoid high tarriffs on this kind of imported good—some things just never change.*

pros when they bought gas, a paper, or a penny bag of sweets. In all, nonmedical suppliers sold about 1.5 million gross a year, at an average price of $10 per gross, for a total of almost $14 million a year. Adjusting for inflation, that is about $140 million in twenty-first-century dollars.

The only place sales figures dropped was at the druggist, where sales accounted for only one-third of all condom sales. They charged an average of $16 per gross, which adds up to $11 million a year. This placed their goods way out of the reach for the average consumer. Besides the higher prices, druggists probably did themselves no favors, remaining the snobs of condom sales and staying away from open display of the little item. Many also forced their clients to ask for their rubbers by name, still insisting on the behind-the-counter, brown-paper-sack method. Still, even though price and availability had a negative impact on the druggists' sales, their profits remained sufficient to "pay the rent" for many pharmacies.

Total condom profits equaled well over $33 million a year. This does not even account for the more than two hundred thousand gross sold to overseas markets (foreign-made condoms were not allowed—legally—into the United States until the 1950s, but American-made condoms were exported to other countries). No wonder that though the top three continued to dominate with about 70 percent of the market share, a handful of smaller manufacturers still vied for a piece of it. In fact, perhaps driven by the fact that there were so few lucrative industries at the time, condom competition was cutthroat, which explains why emphasis was on mass production, not quality control.

FLIPS AND WRINKLES—THE TESTING CONUNDRUM

Casanova would have been proud to know that his inventive ways of assaying his redingotes d'Anglaise had stood the test of time. By the 1930s, there were actually four official methods of mechanical and semimechanical testing used in the United States and one in Great Britain and Germany. In spite of this, though, things had not changed much since the world's greatest lover had entertained his ladies with condom balloons.

The American *flip test* was a labor-intensive, hands-on method. A woman "flipper"—who may not have loved her work or shared what she did with family and friends but was grateful for any kind of employment—sat at a large table with a huge pile of condoms to her left. With her right hand, she hooked one at a time over a pipe connected to a primitive compressor that let out a steady stream of air. When the condom was half full of air, the flipper clamped down in the middle of it and looked for holes or stubborn wrinkles caused by the latex sticking during the vulcanization process.

The flip test was the favorite method of most of the manufacturers who bothered to test at all mainly because it was cheap and there were millions of women willing to do any kind of work for very low pay. It was the Depression. Plus, the ladies were guaranteed a free supply of widows.

Faulty condoms were supposed to be discarded, but this eyes-only method did not eliminate the majority of flawed products making it to market. And most of the major manufacturers who routinely tested had adopted Merle Youngs's method of disposal—sell them to the other guy!

The other techniques used were not much better or terribly different from flipping; there was the *hip test*, where an assembly line tester filled her condoms with air, allowed a sampling to get very large, and then pressed the enlarged condom against her hip or stomach to test for pressure. Sometimes she looked at the balloon for flaws, sometimes not.

The *cheek test* followed the same basic procedure, but the checker held the balloon up to her cheek to feel for air coming through; *cheek II* was the same, but the operator also looked for dirt and other flaws, and was supposed to inflate the samples two times each. More attention to detail. *Cheek II* was considered the most thorough method, and was favored by manufacturers of the best brands.

The English and Germans were far more methodical in their testing; workers, more men than women, inflated each rubber, sealed the end, and placed it on a slow-moving conveyor belt. Any that deflated while traveling across the room fell through a gap in the belt and were swept up and discarded at the end of the day. No seconds for the Europeans.

LEGITIMATE RETAIL

The FDA may have been influenced by the proactive stance taken by states like Oregon, which by 1935, required condoms be sold only through "legitimate" outlets like druggists, jobbers, medical suppliers, directly from manufacturers, or other recognized retail—no more door-to-door sales and the end of vending machines. Retailers of legal condoms in that state had to apply for a license with the state pharmacy board. The guidelines also required some kind of testing, but since there was no money to add condom watchdogs to the state's pharmacy board it is unlikely to have had any real impact on the "illegitimate" sales. The board members also demanded that they personally be supplied with ample samples, leading one witty Oregonian to wonder if perhaps these would be used for party decorations as the authorities celebrated their victory against crummy condoms.

Although consumers had been advised for centuries to use the blow-up test themselves, most men did not bother; others tried to fill their condoms with water to test for holes, but this caused the talcum on them to get sticky, which tended to fill any holes, making it impossible to know if they were flawed or not—and left them looking like a lump of gray bread dough.

And, for all the variety of test methods, it was revealed at the end of the thirties that only about 25 percent of all condoms were exposed to any sort of trial, in the factory or at home.

SEND ME SOME SAMPLES

The incredible success of the condom industry had its downside; its high visibility brought attention to its defects. A biochemist conducting research in 1935 made his findings widely available to the media . . . and to government officials.

Cecil Voge and his research team tested two thousand sheaths, which his assistants purchased from a wide variety of retail outlets around the United States. Blowing up and filling with water every single one of them, Voge found that almost 60 percent of the rubbers were substandard, proving that either there was little testing going on, or the existing methods were inadequate. Since the industrialists were honest in saying that they only tested 25 percent, the numbers were not surprising; and the reluctance on the part of makers to spend the money to test all of their products is not surprising either. Even though labor was cheap, the process slowed the product's journey to market and did add to the cost of production, something that was more significant to the little guys than the major players in the industry. Youngs could afford to do a pretty good job testing his top brand—Trojans—because they fetched premium prices, but he also sold his duds to others.

Because of Voge's very public findings and the fact that the business was so big—it stuck out as a rare example of success in a time of so much failure—in 1937 the Food and Drug Administration decided it was time to get involved in the testing of rubbers.

Ignoring the newly legal "birth control" status of the condom, officials at the FDA decided they could open the doors of the condom producers to the watchful gaze of federal agents by pouncing on its role as disease preventative. The clever administrators declared sheaths were now a drug.

In many ways, the FDA's creativity did have a positive effect on the condom market. Determined to remain ahead of the pack with his Trojan brand—which sold more than thirty million in 1930 alone—Youngs was the first to react and he went so far as to fund the invention of the first genuine technology for advanced testing of each condom manufactured by Youngs Rubber. It was actually the brainchild (and inspired by the European method of testing) of Youngs's brother, who patented his condom-testing conveyor belt in 1940, but it was in use at Youngs's plant by 1938.

In his 1939 description of the new machine, Arthur Youngs explained how after each had been taken from the production conveyor belt, the "article" was placed open end up on a small frame. An automated hose filled it with water. Since the water would come out of any tiny hole or perforation, and was clearly visible to the human eye, defective articles were easy to spot and were removed manually. This eventually proved to be a boon to the big manufacturers of rubbers, saving them a fortune in testing by speeding up the process, cutting down on the number of workers needed for flipping, hipping, or cheeking, and improving the quality tenfold. It also meant that the latex variety had to be finished off without that delicate little dusting of talcum powder.

The FDA's consumer-sensitive regulations had a resounding effect upon the booming industry. For the big boys, it meant a small bite into their profits but it also pushed them into continued modernity, and further market consolidation; to the last of the smaller companies it was the beginning of the end, but it was not the end of federal fiddling.

DEFECTIVE . . . DRUGS?

As if it could get any worse for the smaller manufacturers, Congress unintentionally signed their death warrant when it passed the Food, Drug, and Cosmetic Act of 1938, a bill intended to update and expand the Pure Food and Drug Act of 1906. The new bill, which went into effect in 1940, did not actually mention the condom by name, rather it stated that all drug manufacturers had to guarantee their products to be defect free. Packaging had to include accurate labeling that informed the consumer about who had made the product and where it had been produced, and no incorrect or misleading information could be printed on the package. Before the new legislation, the FDA had the right to keep track of condom testing, but there were no legal mechanisms to assure that every one of the millions sold per year had been tested or to punish abusers if caught. Although Schmid and Youngs chose to follow the letter of the law, others had not. "Condom-as-drug" changed all that.

Immediately after the passage of the new bill, the FDA wasted no time; FDA officials had seized more than six thousand gross defective articles within a month and were confiscating rubbers at an astounding rate. The lawmakers had given the feds a powerful tool to enforce the regulations; not only could they seize any and all crates they knew or assumed were defective, but federal agents also had the power to levy fines against abusers (the law allowed up to ten thousand dollars per seizure). If that was not enough, the federal government could imprison for up to three years anyone who was caught more than once for involvement in the production, transport, or sales of defective items.

Thanks to their use of trademarks and commitment to testing, Schmid, Inc., and Youngs Rubber, both at the top of the heap all along, were the only companies still making legally produced condoms by 1941. Trojans, Sheiks, and Ramses were now the most popular brands in America; they even got the Consumer Union's seal of approval. Sadly, the law said nothing about condoms made for export; even though he had finally seen the error of his ways at home, Youngs continued to sell his seconds overseas. This was also the only legitimate market left for a few of the smaller companies who could not meet FDA standards, but continued to produce for export.

"ADMISSIBILITY OF CONTRACEPTIVE DEVICES"— THE TARIFF ACT OF 1930

Like so much of the history of the condom, it is difficult to reconcile practice with law. By the 1930s, there were still lingering leftovers from the Comstock Act, principally because it had never actually been overturned by Congress, but rather individual court actions had slowly picked away at its impact. One of the remaining leftovers was that birth control could only be sold for medicinal purposes. Women's diaphragms were for prevention of dangerous pregnancies and condoms were for protection against disease. This remaining law clashed directly with the court of appeals decision in 1936 to allow the advertising of sheaths as birth control, not to speak of the open and legal advertising now so common. In shades of Comstock, however, some overzealous federal agents fell back on it in order to prosecute—and persecute—an unsuspecting individual.

Customs agents claiming they took the imports for the purpose of "determining their usefulness for contraceptive purposes," confiscated a large order of pessaries imported from Japan by an American doctor. The District Court for the United States dismissed the suit, declaring that although the statute prohibited "all persons from importing... any article whatever for the prevention of conception," the pessaries were for "proper medical use." The judge went on to declare that as long as birth control items were not imported (or sold) for "immoral reasons," contraceptives "may be manufactured and sold and sent through the mails." A legal expert of the time declared that the Comstock Act had been "almost emasculated by judicial nullification."

In spite of its contribution of one more nail into the coffin of leftover Comstockery, this case illustrates again the strange intersections of morality, the law, the marketplace, and individual choice. Condoms had been used forever for birth control, and it was perfectly legal to sell them as such. Even the military had been promoting them as both disease preventative and birth control—officially! But when preventatives came into the legal spotlight again, the same old morality clause regarding "purpose of use" was trotted out of the closet. Once again, logic and common sense seem to have been absent in the courtroom.

As for the condom industrialists, they just smiled and got on with business.

PRIVATE VERSUS PUBLIC ... AGAIN

In spite of the learning experiences of WWI and the straightforward approach of the Church of England in regard to family limitation, once again private practice and public opinion did not match up with legal or medical practice. Dreadnoughts were selling at a brisk pace, and the British government made condom vending machines illegal (though some townships turned a blind eye to them). The medical community allowed the advertising of sheaths in its journals, but the advertisements were stilted and would not have been read by the general public, making them useless for marketing or educational purposes.

When the National Society for the Prevention of Venereal Diseases attempted to revive the condom as disease preventative by producing The Price of Ignorance, *a short movie dedicated to straightforward education about safe sex, the morality police forced any mention of condoms to be removed, and few publications would even consider printing information on where and when the movie was playing.*

THE SPIRITUAL *DEVICE*

In recognition of the financial reasons to limit family size, in 1931 even the conservative Federal Council of Churches endorsed birth control for "married couples," while at the same time admitting that by doing so, they might be giving the green light for people to indulge in *illicit* sex.

In a similar move across the pond, in 1930 the Lambeth Conference of Bishops of the Anglican Church (the Church of England) reversed its 1920 condemnation of birth control and officially sanctioned its use. Church officials stated that using devices was okay "where there is a clearly-felt moral obligation to limit or avoid parenthood." Dissenters were horrified at the radical move, fearful "artificial means" would lead to having sex anytime, anywhere, which would in turn lead to "selfishness." But the Church of England's leaders showed a very practical side and did not back down from their decision.

Infuriated by such a sinful reversal from the English Church's negative stance on artificial birth control only ten years prior, the Catholic Church

"SEX EDUCATION," DEPRESSION-STYLE

Whether or not Margaret Sanger or her English counterpart, Marie Stopes, had ever read his work is unclear, but it would have been interesting to hear the response of these two women to a sex manual written just for men by George Ryley Scott, published in 1937. This author assured men that it was absolutely necessary for them to control the birth control process—by using condoms—because "Many women are unreliable. The husband cannot be sure that his wife will carry out the requisite technique properly. There are lots of careless women in the world. There are a lot of lazy women. There are a lot of women who are both careless and lazy."

Scott also published The History of Corporal Punishment, *described by one kinky classic bookseller as an "endlessly titillating subject." The author, though, stated in his 1938 treatise that it was to be sold "only . . . to lawyers, sociologists, psychologists," apparently meant to be a serious discovery of all things corporal, including the punishment of children through flagellation, whipping, caning, strapping, and "tawseing" (caning the hands). He followed this up years later with a little favorite titled* Phallic Worship: A History of Sex and Rites.

officially entered for the first time the public debate over contraception. Pope Pius XI issued his encyclical "Casti Connubii" only a few months after the Lambeth conference:

> Since, therefore, openly departing from the uninterrupted Christian tradition some recently have judged it possible solemnly to declare another doctrine regarding this question, the Catholic Church, to whom God has entrusted the defense of the integrity and purity of morals, standing erect in the midst of the moral ruin which surrounds her, in order that she may preserve the chastity of the nuptial union from being defiled by this foul stain, raises her voice in token of her divine ambassadorship and though our mouth proclaims anew: any use whatsoever of matrimony exercised in such a way that the act is deliberately frustrated in its natural power to generate life is an offense against the law of God and of nature, and those who indulge in such are branded with the guilt of a grave sin.

Although the Church had long been against contraception, this is the first time an official statement made it clear that Catholics were not to use anything that would prevent them from "standing erect in the midst of moral ruin"—an interesting turn of phrase given the subject. This stance was to set the stage for Church doctrine for the remainder of the twentieth century and into the twenty-first, since no pope has ever reversed this anti-condom, anti–birth control statement.

The warring church doctrines illuminate a new and very serious schism within the Christian community; and the divide would just get bigger throughout the century, as Catholic doctrine did not mesh with the needs and often the practice of its flock, while more liberal churches like the Anglican began during the Depression to seek ways to help alleviate human suffering by being practical when it came to its parishioners, few of whom could afford big families and too many mouths to feed.

This new struggle would have to wait, however, as the next chapter in the history of the condom was about to begin. And in spite of his hatred of the device, it was Herr Führer who wrote it.

SPAIN AND THE "WHOLLY" *CONDOMINIO*

By the 1930s, the Church had had a major impact on the personal lives of the average Spaniard, which had made buying and using condoms very difficult. In fact, one of the most unlikely uses of one arose directly from the controls of the Church over the Spanish medical community. By this time, scientists had figured out how to count sperm and this made treatment of sterility—at a time and in a culture that worshiped large families—a possibility. The problem was that the Church said that any emission of the seed outside of a woman's body was immoral and illicit. So how to obtain a sample to facilitate identification and treatment for sterility? A "perforated" condom, of course, as described by a leading physician of the day: "When using the perforated condom, let the hole be made in such a way that the majority of the sperm is deposited in the vaginal cavity and only a small amount remains in the condom; otherwise, those maneuvers would be too similar to contraception and would be for that reason illicit."

THIRTEEN

victory . . . will ride on the rubber you save

THE WAR YEARS

As the Second World War began, America was going high tech—CBS and NBC began commercial television transmission in 1941, and Americans *heard* war for the first time as they listened to the attack on Pearl Harbor on their more than thirteen million home radios. Although the United States again entered the European theater late in the game, once committed, American industry took off: Liberty ship, aircraft, vehicle, chemical, and weapon production meant jobs for all—the end of the Depression. But because the need to supply the war effort limited production of consumer goods, there was little difference between the scarcity of the 1930s and that of the war years.

Americans, unlike the British, were new to the concept of rations, but both nations had to put up with shortages and rationing of everything from butter to gas to fabric for new clothes. In response to government calls for personal sacrifices to help the war effort, there were scrap drives held across both countries, collecting all manner of appliances, rags, newspapers, gold, silver, even kitchen grease. And the shortage of rubber was one of the most acute, especially given that with the entry of Japan into the war, access to Indonesian rubber supplies was cut off, leaving the rubber industry hurting.

The pressing demand for rubber in the United States was driven mostly

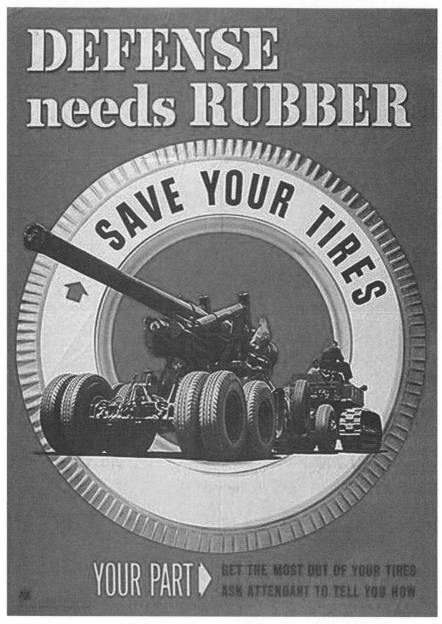

World War II poster: DEFENSE needs RUBBER (but not just for tires!)

by the need to make tires for military vehicles. As the war progressed, the shortage was so extreme that President Roosevelt had to create an Office of Rubber Director to coordinate all production of rubber goods. FDR also asked Americans to donate their household rubber items to be recycled and remade into war materiel. In spite of the "rubber dilemma," though, there was never any suggestion that the condom industry slow down production. Although it was probably a good thing that the millions of avid pro users did not realize that many of their little devices were made from recycled tires, raincoats, garden hoses, shoes, bathing caps, and gloves collected in neighborhood rubber drives, no matter what the source, government officials were determined that there be enough condoms to support the war effort. The lessons of World War I were not forgotten.

Instead of the severe rubber shortage spelling the end for the intrepid condom manufacturers, the production of prophylactics proceeded at a breakneck speed throughout the war, making Schmid and Youngs ever richer, and positioning the London Rubber Company as the sole British producer. No matter the endless shortages, though. In England, where *everything* was rationed, there were two exceptions to the ration rule: beer and condoms. The Home Office defended these exceptions, claiming both were "good for morale."

CONDOM CANCER

Studies done in the late thirties and into the forties proved that employees in British and American rubber factories suffered from increased risk of bladder and other cancers due to their exposure to a variety of harmful chemicals used to prepare rubbers, both the synthetic and the natural varieties. As with the days of brimstoning gut, however, little notice was taken of the health threat to lowly condom workers.

MILITARY SABOTEUR NUMBER ONE

The war definitely proved to American producers that the business of manufacturing condoms could never return to its mom-and-pop roots.

After its initial foray as condom-consumer watchdog in the 1930s, by the 1940s the Food and Drug Administration was joined by the US Public Health Service in an all-out educational effort on the home front. Their singular message to all Americans was simple enough—*use prophylaxis!*

The safe-sex effort, which proved to be very successful, had actually begun in earnest in the 1930s, when FDR had appointed Thomas Parran as surgeon general. Parran was not shy about speaking on the horrors of VD and was responsible for the passage of the National Venereal Disease Control Act of 1938, which was credited with a precipitous drop in the national VD rate by 1940. The spread of sexually transmitted diseases was also checked by the discovery of a strain of penicillin (produced at Oxford University) that was found to be the "easiest" cure yet for syphilis. This medical breakthrough did not slow Dr. Parran's zealous campaign for prophylactic protection, though.

There was also an effort to crack down on prostitution (though Parran remained very vocal about the fact that the military itself was lax in closing down the bordellos that popped up wherever there were men in training)

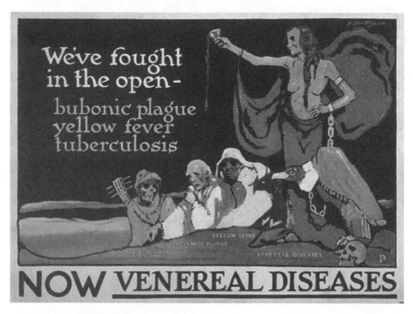

Poster: Social Hygiene Campaign

and the old cry that it was women who spread sexually transmitted diseases was back, with a public education campaign featuring infected females as the "hidden" enemy of freedom and democracy. Even one of history's most famous "cops" got in on the act.

When Eliot Ness, famed organized crime–fighter, joined the Office of Defense Health and Welfare Services at the beginning of the war, he was recruited to use his famous name to make a public statement about his office's efforts against venereal disease. He pointed at prostitutes as the *Military Saboteur Number One*: "That is what health authorities have labeled the 'world's oldest Profession.'" His written address seems stilted and a bit silly by modern standards, but what is most interesting about it is his closing line, intended to assure an anxious public that military policy was wiping out prostitution: "Behind this policy is a record of success in World War I, when the United States mobilized and maintained the least syphilitic army in modern history. With that record in mind, Uncle Sam is not taking camp followers for granted." Mr. Ness was no historian.

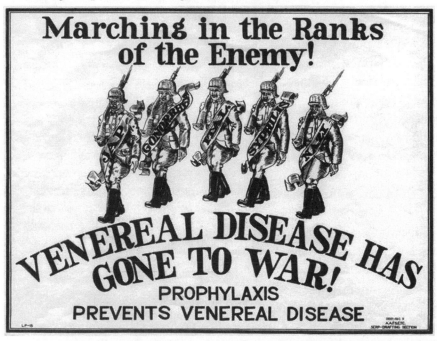

World War II poster: Message to the troops is "Use PROPHYLAXIS!"

If we should have to fight, we should be prepared to do so from the neck up instead of from the neck down.

General James Doolittle, United States Army Air Force

Remember to put it on before you put in!

US Army slogan

Although General Doolittle's remark leaves little doubt about his disapproval of the post–World War I military's approach to disease prevention, the World War II army slogan illustrates that when America entered the Second World War in 1941, the army was ready with an endless supply of "prophey packs" and "pro kits." Army doctors welcomed the bountiful supply, "realizing that angels rightfully belong only in heaven."

Taking advantage of the new technologies available by this time, the military also called upon the advanced technology of moviemaking to produce films to educate soldiers, marines, and sailors about the evils of unprotected sex, one of which spawned yet another popular military slogan: *If you can't say no, take a pro.*

The all-out campaign to educate about VD spawned a pretty wide variety of films produced to help military members understand the need to avoid prostitutes and to use protection no matter whom their partners were. Many of

EVERYONE'S A CRITIC

Though nothing like the concerns voiced during WWI, there were members of the public and some politicians who were as worried about the morals—or lack of—of their military members as they were about their physical safety. The liberal approach to pro distribution and the lascivious films used for instruction were the primary targets of the protesters, leading to the withdrawal of some of the most offensive. But as the brutal war marched on, military leadership was not particularly interested in "moral bleating"; they knew from bitter experience that when men were away from home, and the opportunity arose, soldiers and sailors were going to need more than moral prophylaxis. One angry civilian doctor complained that the army was teaching soldiers about how to use "prophylaxis during sexual misbehavior" instead of teaching them "behavioral control."

the films were very explicit, with plenty of lurid details about how to wear the pro and how to dispose of it when finished. Most GIs called them "Susie

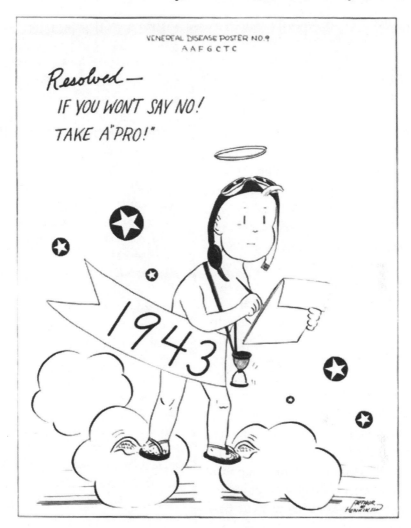

World War II Army Air Force poster

Rotten Crotch" films, but there were those who actually thought they were sexy. Even the films that illustrated what a prophey pack was—these were a staple at boot camp—and how to use it rated high with bored soldiers.

Overall, the visuals employed by the military combining the sexy with the scary worked. Many individual military units actually chose —with the brass's blessings—to use their own slush funds to buy extra supplies of condoms that were made available for free to soldiers and sailors in the barracks and on ships. This policy, along with the strategic placement of vending machines offering a variety of inexpensive sheaths, meant there was no excuse for the men in uniform to go out "unprotected."

Whether or not the soldier-in-training really needed it, no one was allowed off post for more than a few hours of leave without his kit. In fact, by 1942 more than fifty million a month were handed out by the services. That number climbed through to the end of the war, when even at maximum production, the rubber manufacturers had a difficult time meeting the ever-increasing demand.

OVETA CULP HOBBY

Oveta Culp Hobby, born in Killeen, Texas, in 1905, was one of the first women in that state to receive a law degree. She began her amazing career as a member of the Texas House of Representatives, then as an Assistant City Attorney in Houston. She married former Texas governor William P. Hobby, publisher of the Houston Post *and helped him run the newspaper until 1941, when Hobby went to Washington, DC, as head of the war department's Women's Interest Section, a position that paid her a token one dollar a year. She served as director of the WAACs from 1942 to 1945.*

Over 150,000 American women eventually served in what became known as the Women's Army Corps (WAC) and were the first women other than nurses to serve in the ranks of the United States Army.

Hobby was awarded the Distinguished Service Medal for her efforts and after the war she returned to Houston to resume her work at the Post *and to help run a television station her husband had purchased. She returned to Washington, DC, in 1953, when President Dwight D. Eisenhower named her head of the Federal Security Agency, which, later that year, was elevated to a cabinet position and renamed the Department of Health, Education, and Welfare; Hobby was its first secretary.*

THE WACS AND THE WAACS—
NO SLOT MACHINES FOR THESE SOLDIERS

Although many American women had served their country during World War I, they were never given official status or offered a permanent place of their own in the ranks of the US Army. In spite of their devotion to service, the women who worked as ambulance drivers and nurses were "contract workers" and had to fend for themselves, including finding their own billets, food, and medical care. That changed in World War II with the creation of the Women's Army Corps (WACs) and the Women's Army Auxiliary Corps (WAACs), the first all-female military departments in American history.

The corps was the brainchild of one of the few women in power at the time, Congresswoman Edith Nourse of Massachusetts. It was Congresswoman Nourse's intention that any woman who served her country should have the same benefits as the men: her concerns were a direct result of the experiences of those women who had served in the First World War. Nourse's actions were a practical solution to a longtime problem, but the creation of the women's corps did not go as smoothly as she and other supporters like General George Marshall had hoped. The WAACs provided a constant source of gossip within the ranks as well as in the public media, and the debate over women's "proper place" in society raged.

The first director of the WAACs, Colonel Oveta Culp Hobby, understood that she was going to have a difficult sales job, trying to get the American public to understand that women's historic association with the military—mostly as camp followers—was a thing of the past and that they could serve their country honorably as "female soldiers."

Unfortunately, Hobby took a rather Victorian approach when she peddled her "new woman" to the public. Trying not to upset social norms, she characterized her female soldiers as asexual and chaste, an approach that did nothing to prevent rumors spreading about her corps members. Some detractors even accused the government of creating the female corps in order to provide male soldiers prostitutes, making it easy for the military to maintain a "clean" sexual environment. Others did not like the idea of an all-female corps because it would create an ideal breeding ground for lesbianism.

Dismissing it all as nonsense, activist Surgeon General Dr. Parran was interested only in maintaining the health and well-being of all soldiers, and he demanded that the WACs and WAACs be treated as "equals" and issued similar "prophy packs" to those given to male soldiers. Parran even insisted that female soldiers be provided with sex education courses. He also wanted each female latrine to have a fully stocked condom slot machine to provide easy and discreet access.

Busy with her ongoing public relations problems, Hobby rejected off hand all of Parran's demands, citing public doubts and accusations, which she believed would get worse if her soldiers were issued prophylactics. Her answer to sex education was to hand an "educational" booklet to each female officer, whose job it was to preach and teach abstinence and chastity to her troops. Perhaps the lessons of World War I were not applicable to military women.

UNCLE SAM'S CONTRACEPTIVES

Hobby's approach did not prevent the "whispering campaign" that began in 1943, fueled by articles written by John O'Donnell of the *New York Daily News*. He told readers that the WAACs deployed overseas were being issued pros as birth control, which led to a huge public outcry. After a brief official investigation found that the rumors had been started by male servicemen angry about women making inroads into the once man-only environment (taking over "cushy" office jobs, forcing the former occupants closer to the front), Secretary of War Henry Stimson, General Marshall, and Colonel Hobby all agreed that they would have to declare all such claims blatant lies. But the public actually seemed to find another source of denial much more compelling.

When Ruth Gowan, an Associated Press correspondent based in North Africa where many WAACs served, wrote, "If Uncle Sam handed out contraceptives, I got left out. And I understood I was to be issued the same equipment as the WAACs," her readers loved it. Other pro-WAAC reporters were far more serious in their tones, castigating their rumormongering peers as sensationalist, even sexist.

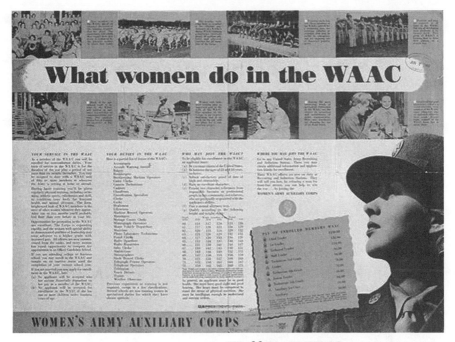

World War II WAAC recruitment poster

As hard as Hobby and the supportive members of the press tried, though, no one could tap down all the gossip, as evidenced by the report of an army investigator at a post in Kansas City; he chronicled that members of the public believed that the "WAACs were issued condoms and enrolled solely for the soldier's entertainment, serving as 'morale builders' for the men and nothing more." Nor could she or her superiors force newspapers to stop yellow press–style headlines like "Stork Pays Visit to WAAC Nine Days after Enlistment" and "Army Officer Tried for Bigamy."

DEAR DORAS AND AGONY AUNTS— THE DOROTHY DIXES OF CONDOMS

It was not just governments that provided information about sex and prevention. Women's magazines, which had become very popular in the

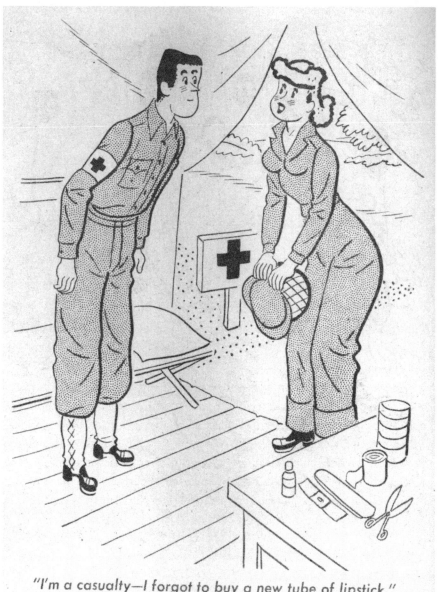

"I'm a casualty—I forgot to buy a new tube of lipstick."

Winnie the WAC cartoons

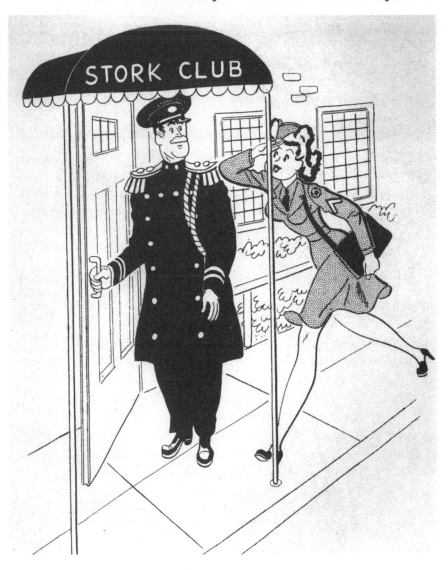

United States and the United Kingdom by the 1920s, enjoyed a wide readership during the war and owed a large part of their popularity to the question-and-answer sections called the Dorothy Dix pages. Advice column journalist Elizabeth Gilmer, who wrote under the pseudonym "Dorothy Dix," was supposed to have originated the idea and her name stuck.

Although it was a very quiet process, by the 1940s the Dorothy Dix pages (later called Dear Doras and Agony Aunts) of many popular women's magazines had become an important source of information about sex and sexual matters. Many people were hungry to understand and solve sexual problems, but were too embarrassed to ask friends, family, or their doctors. The appearance of advice columnists had ushered in a sort of underground public education program, unsponsored by any ham-handed government agency—and they sold magazines, which made these columnists very popular with publishers who turned a blind eye to the more blatant subjects discussed.

In the United States, medical expert Karl Menninger combined an Agony Aunts–style advice column with user-friendly medical information. In Britain and Australia, the same kind of advice was meted out by Norman Haire, a pioneer in sexual pedagogy. Both men recommended different birth control devices, including condoms, and their columns were even popular with soldiers, who found this form of delivery about "avoiding diseases while in uniform" very informative and more interesting than the coarse way in which their sergeants and officers jammed the safe-sex message down their throats. This must have provided an interesting vignette, the tough soldier propped up on his cot reading a magazine whose front cover promised to reveal all the secrets of the season's latest hairstyles and how to bake a cake without using eggs.

Interestingly, though these sex advice columnists received little public critique or criticism for their candidly written opinions, that changed when it was tried on the radio. Talk show hosts who were sex experts invited listeners to call in with their questions about anything sexual or highly personal in nature; this is the birthplace of a format still popular today in radio. Though the ban on mentioning words like *sex* on the radio was lifted in the United States and England in the early forties, when the audio version of the Dorothy Dix pages first aired, public opinion turned against the sex experts—mostly due to the fact that anyone could listen, and the medical information given out could corrupt young children and seniors. So, the condom got little play over the radio, but in women's magazines, it did all right.

> ## THE LYCEUMS OF THE FORTIES
> *Some of the advice columnists took advantage of the wave of interest in attending sex lectures by offering themselves to local groups as experts in the subject. Guests would either ask a question out loud, or submit their questions in writing. These ran the gamut from whether a "genital kiss" was perverted to whether condom use was "decent" as a "marital device."*

OVERPAID, OVERFED, OVERSEXED, AND OVER HERE

It did not take long after arriving on British soil in 1942 for American GIs to gain the reputation of being sex-mad; plenty of British women were very attracted to them. British men were also off fighting in all corners of the globe, for years at a time, leaving young women to fend for themselves and to seek company and romance with foreigners.

There were of course girls like the "Piccadilly Warriors"—amateur prostitutes supplementing meager factory wages or just making a bit of extra cash on the side—who were paid for their services. But most relationships between GIs and British women were not businesslike, unless chocolate bars and hose can be counted.

Some of the reasons British women gave for their attraction to American men included the American uniforms, which were more complimentary than the British; that the American soldier and sailor earned three times as much as their British counterparts; because most Americans had access to rationed goods; and, they were jovial . . . and available, with more than three million swarming over the island nation by D day in 1943. And the Americans lived up to their reputations—even American officers admitted that their men were sex-obsessed, a fact perfectly expressed by one US soldier: ". . . army conversation has a beautiful simplicity and directness. It is all on one solid, everlasting subject . . . Women, Women, Women."

And though the behaviors of predatory American soldiers and some English women shocked many Britons, there had been a lessening of traditional norms going on for many generations, and guilt did not accompany busy sex lives. After the war, one British housewife summed it all up with

"We were not really immoral, there was a war on." This attitude was also evident in Europe.

TOO MUCH TIME ON THEIR HANDS

Although estimates vary, military history experts generally agree that the average GI who served in Europe from D day to the end of the war had sex with about twenty-five women. By the time Germany surrendered, the US occupying army had to ration condoms to four per soldier per month, something an army official complained was "entirely inadequate." A 1945 US Army survey documented that "the level of promiscuity among the troops was far higher than officially admitted, and rates rose in direct proportion to the amount of time the men had spent overseas."

When the American military occupied Italy, it was estimated that 75 percent of all soldiers had sex regularly with Italian women. In spite of their availability, though, fewer than half of those liaisons involved the use of condoms. But the most active American military men, sexually speaking, were black GIs, who were even more likely to have had sex while serving in Europe. Unfortunately, these soldiers trained and functioned in segregated units and were less likely to have been exposed to the condom message by their superiors. Many of those who were educated about protection reported that they felt pros robbed a man of his "virility," perhaps the most likely reason why these troops suffered a much higher incidence of VD.

CHAPLAIN'S COMPLAINTS

The American Catholic hierarchy never committed sufficient chaplains to join the military in the European or Pacific theaters, and burnout in the priests' ranks was a huge problem. That did not stop them, however, from constantly complaining and preaching against the army's willingness to provide "inappropriate" reading material—cheap illustrated magazines with pinup girls—but especially against the "easy access to condoms" policy. Even in the middle of a battlefield, chaplains found every chance to preach against the "venury of the condom." One such chaplain stationed in England was positively vociferous about it, but probably wished later he'd heeded the message to use pros—he discovered that after an affair with an English woman he ended up with VD.

"V" FOR VICTORY GIRLS

British and European women were not the only ones who were exceptionally sexually active during the war. Much like the "Khaki fever" of World War I, when young American women threw themselves at men in uniform, as the Second World War began many young women (including teenagers) offered themselves to any man in uniform. They were dubbed the "Victory Girls," "Khacki-wachies," and "good-time Charlottes." Unlike the Europeans, these women simply enjoyed the excitement of treating a soldier or sailor to sex without ties. It also appears from the unplanned pregnancy and VD rates of the time that while at home at least, the men

A NIGHT AT THE OPERA

After Allied troops had marched into Italy, some had the opportunity to experience a little of the local color of the Italian towns, cities, and villages they occupied. In the lovely town of Bari, which boasted a beautiful opera house, there was a night at the opera that those in attendance likely never forgot. During a performance of The Merry Widow, a soldier sitting high up in the balcony stood up, unnoticed, and blew up a condom to enormous size, tied it off, and let it float down into the audience below. Though many pairs of eyes were on the big balloon, like the nine-hundred-pound gorilla in the living room, no one acknowledged its presence, until an annoyed nurse pushed it away; others followed suit, and began punching it up into the air. Meanwhile, soldiers all over the opera house were blowing up their rubbers and tossing them into the air, until the staid opera environment had turned into a circus, but one that had everyone laughing. Perhaps it was the name of the opera that inspired the first soldier to induce such inappropriate behavior.

(and women) did not use condoms very often, perhaps because the young women would have had little or no exposure to the safe-sex message and the men felt their instant paramours were so young, they were "clean."

It did not take long for these quickie liaisons to come to the attention of military leaders, and the army soon turned its attention to teaching soldiers that these young women might have looked like the girl next door, but it was GI BEWARE. With what was probably the most widely distributed pamphlet of the war, a publication featuring a fresh-faced girl titled *She Looked Clean—But . . .* was found at every US military facility around the world. It is interesting to note that once again the woman was blamed for

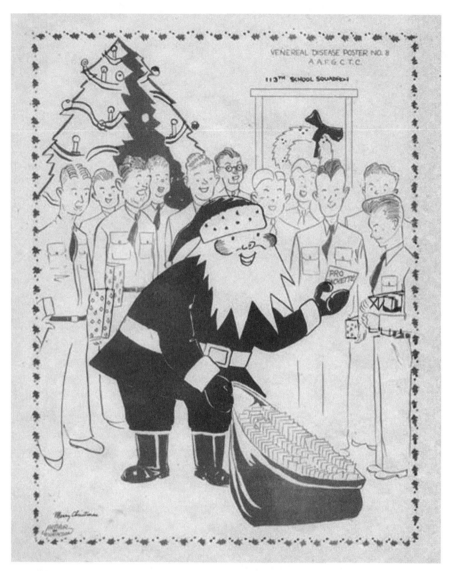

World War II Army Air Force poster: Santa delivering the pros

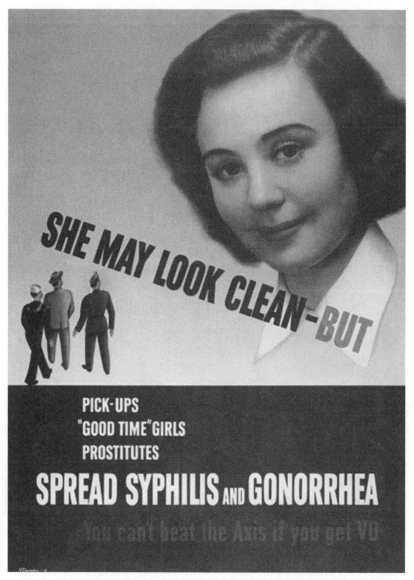

World War II VD education pamphlet

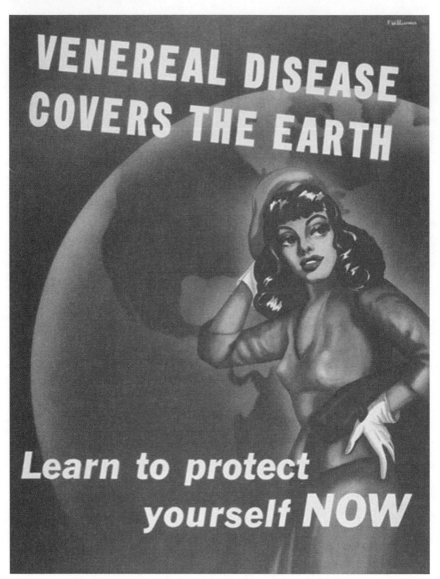

World War II US public education poster

promiscuity and ensuing disease. No one ever suggested that it might be wise to warn the girls that soldiers might be infected, nor was the GI ever blamed for his part in the "act."

PATENTED ARTICLES

English patent law officials had always shown a strong prejudice toward condom production because "these are not articles for which . . . the Crown can be expected to exercise its discretion by way of granting a patent," making manufacturers somewhat reluctant to invest a great deal in domestic production, preferring to purchase German-made rubbers and stamping English names on the imports. That changed when the London Rubber Company decided to go high tech and, patent or no, geared up for mass production just prior to the war. Company executives spent a lot of money to employ highly mechanized production methods that put them in the perfect position to get the only government contract in the early forties intended to supply the British army and navy, along with some of the American soldiers stationed in England, with their Dreadnoughts. London Rubber was cranking out more than thirty-six million per year throughout the war.

But the English company could not possibly keep up with the world-wide demand. It was no surprise that Schmid and Youngs met the challenge of not only supplementing British production, but when it could be managed, they even shipped to other European nations, as well as the beleaguered Russians.

KAUTSCHUCKS AND *GUMMIS* . . . HITLER'S HATRED OF THE CONDOM

Very early in their march toward absolute power, Nazi party officials insisted that sexuality, reproduction, and marriage were all related and could not be separated in order to meet momentary carnal desires, which were injurious to the health and well-being of the country as a whole.

Beginning right after the Nazi takeover of Germany in 1933, a series of laws was passed in an attempt to officially control German access to birth control. Heinrich Himmler ordered that only pharmacies could sell preventatives, and they could only be wrapped in plain brown wrappers. No more of the decorative, eye-catching packaging that had caught on by the end of the 1920s and could be found in German pharmacies, barbershops, open-air markets, brothels, and other retail outlets. And certainly no more labels making it clear that what was in the ugly brown packages remained a handy birth control device.

By the late 1930s, well-known Nazi physician and author Ferdinand Hoffman documented that what was being preached by the regime was not what was being practiced by young Germans. A typical Nazi, this condom-hater had no problem finding Jews at fault for the popularity of the *Kautschuck*. He blamed the high incidence of premarital sex among young Germans on Jewish doctors who Hoffman said not only provided condoms and other birth control to patients, but even educated both men and women about sexuality—and its "pleasures." He described in disgust how young people "parked" in cars in "the woods ... where so-called love is made." Yes, said Hoffman, it was because of those Jewish doctors that Germans were using more than seventy-two million condoms a year by the time the war began. (Nazis also referred to syphilis as the "Jewish disease.")

Hoffman's anti-Semitic nonsense did not, of course, reflect the true history of the German condom. Prior and immediately after World War I, Germany was the condom capital of Europe. Since the late nineteenth century, the German military had been vigorous in making *gummis* available to all sailors and soldiers for the prevention of venereal diseases. The civilian population had been using them for even longer, but as birth control. It was war that stopped the international commerce, but it did not stop their production for domestic use.

The internal condom war raged for years within the Nazi Party itself, with the "pro-condom/anti-VD" side winning against those who were sure that many naughty Germans were cheating and using the disease preventatives for other purposes. Out of concern over the spread of disease, there continued to be easy-to-find vending machines all over Germany.

The condomites continued to prevail until the end of 1941, when the

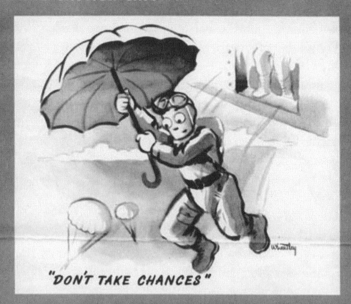

poster child for sexual ambivalence, Adolph Hitler, finally put his foot down and ordered a total ban on all birth control—an order that coincided with a natural curtailment of condom distribution caused by an acute shortage of natural rubber, which led to the eventual discovery by the Germans of a synthetic variety. His concern was not one of morality but because he was worried that German women were not reproducing sufficient amounts of new Nazis to replace those who were dying in war. Despite the absolute ban and the rubber shortage, though, the German military continued to be supplied with gummis up to the bitter end. Hitler showed a very practical side when he insisted that his elite troops be supplied with plenty of *kautschucks* in order to "preserve" their ability to fight.

IL DUCE'S *PROFILATTICOS*

Similar to the Nazi efforts to control German sexuality, Italian Fascist leader Benito Mussolini and his followers had been trying since the 1920s to make birth control of any sort absolutely illegal. By the late twenties, his Law for Public Safety made writing about and distributing information about contraception a punishable offense: the production, advertising, and selling of *profilatticos* was strictly outlawed. Mussolini's efforts were not driven by any religious or moralistic concern for his fellow Italians. He and his followers were worried about the birthrate, which had been dropping since the late nineteenth century. By the war years, this drop in population left the Fascists—like their Nazi counterparts—wondering if there would be anyone left to man the army and farm the fields. They were so determined to get Italians to reproduce, secondary laws were passed, carrying harsh punishments for anyone who defied the public safety bans. What amounted to sex police were employed to patrol the chemist shops and open-air markets to try to root out anyone who might be buying and selling wares illegally.

Il Duce did not stop at that, though. He was so determined to boost the population, he came up with his "populationist" strategy, which included the Bachelor Tax. This penalized any man between the age of twenty-five to sixty-five if he remained unmarried, apparently assuming that only married men "helped" with reproduction. The tax was handy in a way, since it ended up funding all the new orphanages necessary because of the huge increase in abandoned children the government had to care for, a result of the new laws banning condoms.

No matter how many sex police or fines were levied, however, concern over contracting venereal disease remained, and throughout the war years, Italians did have limited and highly controlled access to condoms as *preservativos*. True to the history of the little device, though, Italians defied the laws and their grand leader: black marketeers profited nicely from selling high-quality condoms—as birth control.

NEITHER CONTRACEPTION NOR PREVENTATIVE . . . THE CREATIVE CONDOM

While British inventors were developing *Colossus*, the ultimate code-breaking machine, which cracked the vital German "Enigma" code, the condom was inspiring innovation within the ranks. In displays of great ingenuity, as men crossed the English Channel toward Dunkirk and Normandy, American soldiers used rubbers to keep their guns and ammunition dry. American radio operators making the rough journey in the lumbering, wet Amtanks improvised covers to keep their microphones dry—condoms were the perfect fit. British soldiers and sailors who were stationed along coastal areas where moisture was a constant problem for equipment had made the

BULLET HOLES AND WATER BALLOONS

After being shot in the chest, a young soldier woke up to find the holes in his chest plugged with condoms to stop the bleeding. Other soldiers and airmen flying over Germany found them handy as portable loos, filling them up and sending them out the cargo doors of planes, a little present for the Nazis below.

NEIGHBORHOOD LEGEND

There was a story going around during the war that a British soldier's use of his prophy to keep his gun's firing mechanism warm in freezing weather led to the suggestion that Durex manufacture eighteen-inch condoms; Churchill was said to have agreed on two conditions—that the condom be labeled "Made in Britain," and "Medium."

same discovery. It was even suggested that condom manufacturers make fifteen- to eighteen-inchers, which would have been perfect for the big guns and other vulnerable equipment. Schmid, it seems, never got the message.

Probably the most creative nonsexual use of prophylaxis, though, was the brainchild of a group of British propagandists who desperately needed to figure out how to drop propaganda messages over Germany during the rainy season. One of these clever—or desperate—folks came up with the idea of poking the messages intended for German civilians into condoms, then inflating them so that they would float gently to the ground. These were loaded onto aircraft and released over major city centers. There is no way to know whether the population made any practical use of the deliveries.

THE PACIFIC THEATER...
BLACK PROPAGANDA IN THE PHILIPPINES

Far darker than the novel use of prophylaxis for the delivery of propaganda, military PSYOP (psychological operations) campaigns, waged by both the Allies and the Axis, were not above using fear of venereal disease to try to influence the opinions of indigenous peoples. Preceding the American military arrival to the Philippines, the Japanese waged a PSYOP campaign to convince Filipinos that Americans considered

> ## PROTESTING BLUES
> *Protesting the insult to their manhood after higher authorities tried to limit their exposure to venereal disease by requiring they use prophylactics, the elite troops of the Spanish "Blue Division" stationed along the Eastern Front affixed inflated condoms to their bayonets as they marched in review for a contingent of very senior German officers.*

their women little more than prostitutes. In a twisted attempt to turn the islanders against Americans, the Japanese dropped leaflets written to look like they had been printed by and for the American military, warning GIs to protect themselves against the diseases local women carried:

Guard against Venereal Disease

Lately there has been a great increase in the number of venereal diseases among our officers and men owing to prolific contacts with Filipino women of dubious character. Due to hard time and stricken conditions brought about by the Japanese occupation of the islands, Filipino women are willing to offer themselves for a small amount of foodstuffs. It is advisable in such cases to take full protective measures by use of condoms, protective medicines . . . better still to hold intercourse only with wives, virgins, or women of respective character. Furthermore, in view of the increase in pro-American leanings, many Filipino women are more than willing to offer themselves to American soldiers and due to the fact that Filipinos have no knowledge of hygiene, disease carriers are rampant and due care must be taken.

Considering how many dialects were spoken on the islands, and the fact that very few locals were literate, in English or otherwise, it is unlikely the complex messages had the intended effect.

THE SADDEST SIDE OF CONDOM USE

Reminiscent of the German and Slavic military-run brothels of World War I, beginning in the 1930s the Japanese military bought and kidnapped thousands, probably hundreds of thousands, of girls to work as "comfort women" for Japanese soldiers and officers. Many of these women were forced to work in makeshift facilities very near the dangerous front lines.

JAPANESE ATTACKS

The primary producer of Japanese military condoms was the Kokusia Rubber Company, known today as Okamoto Rubber Manufacturing Company and founded in 1934. This company is under attack by women's groups in Japan because of one of its brand names: the Attack Champion has been condemned as a gross and inappropriate throwback to the ugly history of condom use by soldiers and seamen who used the forced services of so many enslaved women.

Okamoto USA, Inc., located in Stratford, Connecticut, markets more subtly named products like Beyond Seven and Crown Condoms.

The "Senso Daughters," or "daughters of war," came from mostly Asian countries, including East Timor, China, the Philippines, Formosa (Taiwan), Indonesia, as well as the West Indies, but the majority were from Korea. There are no reliable figures as to how many women were forced into service as military prostitutes—in part because as they were shipped to wherever they were deemed necessary, and shipping manifests listed them as numbered cargo, not by their names—but some experts on the subject estimate that as many as three hundred thousand women suffered this fate.

The Japanese military imposed rules for all "comfort stations," and one of those rules was that the men had to use condoms. A typical sign at the entrance of a station read:

- This brothel does not admit anyone other than army soldiers . . . visitors are required to show their brothel permit.
- Visitors must pay service charges at the reception counter and in return receive an entrance ticket and a condom.
- Service charges are as follows: 2 yen for noncommissioned officers, soldiers, and civilian employees . . .
- Those having bought a ticket may enter the designated room, with a time limit of 30 minutes.
- The ticket should be handed to the ianfu [comfort woman] upon entering the room.
- When finished, leave the room quickly.
- Those violating rules or disturbing military morals will be forced to leave.
- Do not touch ianfu without a condom.

Years after the horrors they had endured were still a grim memory, many of the women recalled that the most degrading job at the comfort stations was that of cleaning the condoms at the end of the day. Although the supplies of *Attack 1* (since they were military issue, they were labeled with military designations) were plentiful, there were areas in the massive Pacific front that suffered from shortages, and condoms were used over and over again.

I'M GOING FRATTIN' AND FEAR OF THE FURLOUGH . . . AMERICAN SOLDIERS CAN'T GO HOME

When the war was at an end and there were still hundreds of thousands of American troops stationed in Europe, it meant that there were a lot of bored soldiers looking for fun. Recognizing the possible dangers inherent in lots of idle hands and minds, the military stepped up its efforts to try to keep pent-up soldiers seeking solace and entertainment—sex—from contracting VD. Educational posters were cheap to produce and easy to ship, and reappeared at all military facilities throughout Europe. One of the most common featured a sad GI on his cot, head hung low. The caption read, "VD—a sorry ending to a furlough. Prophylaxis prevents venereal disease!"

Strangely, in spite of all the public and military sex education and freely available preventatives, the occupation army in postwar Germany had the highest rate of venereal disease since that of the doughboys. The problem was manyfold: German women were so poor that freelance prostitution was a way to survive the extreme poverty postwar Germans experienced and the American military was stretched too thin to police its own. This meant women who had survived the hardships imposed by war, and cared (or knew) little about sexual hygiene, were passed from man to man. It also

ARMY REPORT ON SEX EDUCATION IN THE MILITARY
A record of the medical problems of one US Army unit stated:

This unit scheduled lectures by the battalion surgeon or exhibitions of venereal disease prevention training films twice a month. Company commanders lectured on sex hygiene once a month. Platoon sergeants also lectured once a month. For purposes of dispelling fear of prophylaxis treatment, demonstration prophylaxis was given in every squad of the organization. Mechanical prophylaxis kits were supplied to every man going on pass. Individual kits were given to each man going on overnight pass or furlough. Each man returning from pass was required to report to the dispensary and state whether or not he needed prophylactic treatment. The location of prophylactic stations was posted in every barrack. Posters advertising the value of prophylaxis were widely displayed.

appears to have been a time when many soldiers had become overly confident in the new penicillin treatments readily available from medics and doctors, leading them to ignore the constant warnings to wear condoms. Whatever their reasons, some servicemen took their chances.

Once the military faced the fact that the VD epidemic in postwar Germany had to be dealt with, they revamped some of their VD rules. In order to make sure soldiers who were infected would come in for treatment instead of continuing to spread disease, a longtime policy of punishing those found infected was lifted and soldiers who had had unsafe sex were encouraged to go to their medics for a Wasserman test and treatment. The army aggressively passed out V-Packettes (V for Victory) to all soldiers; these included condoms and chemical treatments. Lots of prophylactic distribution points were set up at Red Cross clubs and train stations throughout the American occupation zone

THE INCREDIBLE *PRO*?

Stan Lee, famous for his cartoon characters the Incredible Hulk and Spider-Man, also lent his talents to a somewhat earthier cause.

But at any rate I was asked to do a poster that would admonish the enlisted men, saying every time they had done the wild thing with a girl overseas, they should go to one of the "prophylactics stations," which dotted the landscape in Europe. Set up by the army, they were little places with a green light above the door. When you walked in there, they did terrible things, which I don't even want to think about—but which apparently cured you, or prevented you from getting an incurable disease. At any rate it was like mission impossible. My assignment, if I would accept it, was to do this poster that would warn the soldiers to go to these little "pro stations." I thought: "What on Earth could I do?" Then finally I drew a little cartoon figure of a soldier walking through a door with a green light above it. He looks very smug and self-satisfied, and a dialogue balloon above his head said "VD? Not me!" They must have printed a hundred trillion of those things. So in my own humble way, I think I probably won the war single-handedly, because if that stopped them from getting ill then they were all ready and set to fight. And that's the untold story of how we won the war.

where soldiers could get as many pros as they needed. They were also asked to read the pamphlets that were handed out by volunteers explaining proper condom handling; these even included how to dispose of the items, in order to assure they would not be recycled.

There was no hint of the old World War I moral prophylaxis. Soldiers were simply asked to protect themselves from infection, no questions asked. The military also took its men's "needs" seriously by vetting brothels that agreed to allow American doctors to test their prostitutes. When a facility passed the test, it was put on a list of best places to frequent. Judging by the long lines at the American Army–controlled brothels, the plan worked.

THE BABY BOOM!

When the war came to an end, tens of millions of military men and women, along with untold numbers of civilians, had been killed. The world was changed forever. But despite the horrors wrought by war, one thing is certain; in spite of what they had seen in combat, and despite the amazing rates of sex the boys had had while away, when they came home, they were "ready." In 1945 and 1946, both the British and the American marriage rates exploded—as did birthrates. Especially the American.

In 1945, there were 2,873,000 babies born in the United States; in 1946, 3,500,000, a 20 percent increase in just one year. That fact, taken with the emergence of "miracle" drugs that meant fewer and fewer people felt compelled to use condoms to protect themselves from VD—they were almost obsolete as prophylaxis by 1960—would lead one to think that the firms of Schmid and Youngs should finally have realized their own Black Friday after the war. Instead, contrary to the booming birthrate, most sexually active Americans continued to use condoms when they wanted to practice birth control.

Strangely, and not for the last time, it was the military that did an about-face when it came to pro use. By 1947, in what sounded like a repeat of the moral prophylaxis of the 1910s, the American army embarked on a "character" education program that reversed the wartime philosophy of "protection was paramount." Now, any lectures delivered on sexual health and well-being were to be one hour in duration, and only ten minutes of that time could be used to discuss prophylaxis. And, in that discussion the limitations of condom use were emphasized, not the benefits. The old rules about punishing someone for contracting VD were back, too. Any man diagnosed lost his leave and would not be recommended for promotion—ever.

Back was the old cry that teaching GIs how to protect themselves—except by practicing abstinence—was promoting "venery" and "safeguarding promiscuity."

No more "Putting it on before putting it in."

FOURTEEN

backseat bingo with my classy chassis . . . let's get it on!

FROM BABY BOOM TO MODERN PLAGUE

*O*nly a few years after the end of the war, former soldiers and their growing families were using the GI Bill to buy cookie-cutter homes in new suburbs like Levittown, New York. By 1948, Californians could take a drive to eat their first McDonald's hamburger. Soon after, Americans were tuning in to Ed Sullivan's variety show on their more than fifteen million television sets, while anyone could enjoy a vacation across country, staying in that new chain of motor hotels called the Holiday Inn.

Women were back at home, trading in their uniforms and overalls for feminine dresses and perfectly coiffed hair, while magazine and television ads sent the message that to be a "real woman," she had to cater to her husband and family—after all, what could be more important than experimenting with over one hundred Jell-O recipes! It did not take long for Rosie the Riveter to became a distant memory.

In Britain the picture was not much different; the brave women of war became mums and wives once again, and after so many years of deprivation, the American model of consumerism and label consciousness was quickly adopted. The sale of cars exploded, as did that of most manufactured goods. Young men and women also enjoyed Coke along with the lessening of class restraints, which meant a lot more social mobility. The war had dealt the final blow to the old social order.

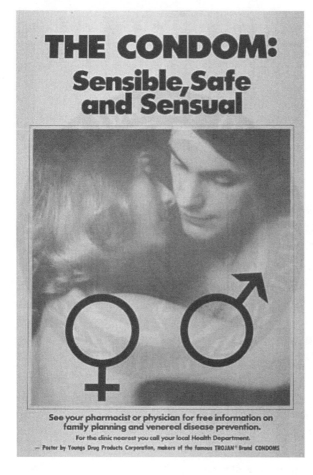

Trojan-sponsored poster campaign

In spite of the public objectification of women as household icons and perfect mothers, and Lucy and Desi sleeping in separate beds, Americans were not as chaste as they have so often been portrayed in potted histories of the 1950s. While many may have been cocooning in an attempt to be normal again, the postwar period was actually a sexy era. Marilyn Monroe was strutting her stuff on screen and off—she was the first to pose for the cover of Hugh Hefner's new magazine, *Playboy*—and "Elvis the Pelvis" was gyrating his way into young women's hearts while he introduced a brand-new, often-controversial music genre ... *rock and roll* was here to stay.

It is perhaps the novel, however, that documents the discrepancies in the sexual mores of the time: *Peyton Place*, with everything from adultery to premarital sex, was the most read book of the decade and revealed that age-old hypocrisy, the clash between public chastity versus sex in the real world.

The truth about American lifestyles was also documented in the controversial *Kinsey Report*, which literally proved men and women were

HOW TO HAVE A HAPPY HUSBAND
From a 1950s high school, home economics textbook

Have dinner ready. Plan ahead, even the night before, to have a delicious meal—on time. This is a way of letting him know that you have been thinking about him and are concerned about his needs. Most men are hungry when they come home, and the prospect of a good meal is part of this warm welcome needed.

Prepare yourself. Take 15 minutes to rest so that you'll be refreshed when he arrives. Touch up your makeup, put a ribbon in your hair and be fresh-looking. He has just been with a lot of work-weary people.

Be a little gay and a little more interesting. His boring day may need a lift.

Clear away the clutter. Make one last trip through the main part of the house just before your husband arrives gathering up school books, toys, paper, etc. Then run a dust cloth over the tables. Light a candle. Your husband will feel he has reached a haven of rest and order, and it will give you a lift, too.

Prepare the children. Take a few minutes to wash the children's hands and faces (if they are small), comb their hair, and if necessary, change their clothes. They are little treasures and he would like to see them playing the part.

Minimize all noise. At the time of his arrival, eliminate all noise of the washer, dryer, dishwasher or vacuum. Try to encourage the children to be quiet. Better yet, have them in bed.

enjoying sex *a lot*. Statistically, American women of the fifties had sex far more often than women of the twenty-first century. The same held true for Britons, who were studied in the "Little Kinsey" report, the difference being they remained more restrained in their public behaviors and sex stayed behind closed doors.

In the medical community, there were some well-known names who spoke out about sexual repression as an "un-healthful condition"; famous psychiatrists like Carl Rogers and Eric Fromm warned that ignoring the libido was dangerous and what people needed to do was relax and accept their very human drives and impulses, which would in turn lead to happier, healthier lives. This message was even carried by the conservative Norman Vincent Peale, who warned about the dangers of repressing sexual appetites. America's favorite pediatrician, Dr. Spock, got into the act when he assured worried parents that when their young children masturbated, it was nothing to become alarmed over.

> ## "SEXUAL BEHAVIOR OF THE HUMAN MALE/FEMALE"
> *When Alfred Kinsey's controversial studies were published in 1948, they proved again how hungry individual Americans were for information about their own bodies, drives, and sex in general. The books got lots of praise and lots of criticism and they certainly proved what the humble little condom had "known" for centuries—public beliefs and private behaviors rarely correspond.*

> ## ROCKING
> *The term* rocking *began as a expression meant to refer to the physical movements gospel singers made while "rocking in their souls" with Jesus. But in the late forties when a blues singer, Roy Brown, wrote the song "Good Rocking Tonight," a parody on gospel, rocking became a widely understood euphemism for sex. Within the African American community, the term had had double meaning since the twenties, but by the fifties "everybody understood" and many were offended when the term* rock and roll *was coined, convinced it was capitalizing on "that other" meaning.*

Legally speaking, the antiquated Comstock statutes that remained in a handful of states continued to fade away. Only Massachusetts and Connecticut retained laws that limited where and how condoms and other birth control devices could be sold (although more than thirty states prohibited retailers from advertising their products as birth control).

By 1955 thousands of medical personnel were receiving formal training on best practice in family planning at the many Planned Parenthood clinics that continued to pop up around the country.

In fact, as new conflicts were appearing all over the world, as the cold war and the Korean War began, and as the French were being defeated in Vietnam, condom manufacturers were doing very well indeed.

THE FDA'S SUCCESSES

As much of an irritant as the FDA had been to the condom industry, the big manufacturers owed that agency a large debt of gratitude. Without government interference, the condom would have remained a fairly primitive instrument, never moving beyond the bad old days of pesky holes and questionable quality.

By the fifties, though, standardization had paid off. Manufacturers were able to meet increasingly stringent requirements, which along with the fast-paced growth of retail chains enhanced sales. Suburbanization meant Americans were spreading across the country, and where there were new suburbs there were bigger and better retail chains right behind. Drug stores popped up everywhere, and the chain stores were not shy about putting up colorful displays selling an increasing variety of rubbers. Along with this increased visibility came new kinds of marketing strategies; with easier access, pilferage became a problem and chain stores had to devise new ways of displaying their goods, making sure not to put too many packages out at a time—stealing condoms in quantity had become quite the thing, especially with teenaged boys.

Prior to 1957, the same year the English brand Durex introduced lubricated sheaths, American import laws relaxed, and for the first time foreign-made condoms could be sold on the US market. The British were the first to take advantage of that change by bringing lubricated condoms onto the American market, soon to be copied by their US counterparts. Though the British had gone far to produce comfortable and disposable condoms, it was still possible to buy the ever-durable, meant-to-be-reused Paragon long after the war. By all reports, one had to *be* a paragon to put up with the thick, inflexible device just for the sake of saving a few schillings.

But the comfortable life of the humble little condom was about to change—again—beginning with the reemergence of an old ally and sometimes friend.

Margaret Sanger, America's birth control icon, was a fragile little old lady in her seventies when she returned to the birth control fold, making her last and, some might argue, biggest impact on American sexuality, realizing her lifelong dream of putting birth control solely in the hands of women. Enter the *Pill*.

A "MAGIC LITTLE PILL"

Although her efforts on behalf of women to allow them to take control over their own bodies had led to the slow but steady erosion of the Comstock

Act, Sanger was never completely satisfied with the way things had gone. Although she had given her tacit support for the use of condoms, the complaint about putting all the power in the hands of men had never gone away; and the scientific community considered research on birth control a taboo. This left the free market to simply continue to produce variations on the same theme: messy topical creams, cumbersome diaphragms, and primitive IUDs, many of which were not only uncomfortable but could be dangerous to a woman's health. There was also a significant rise in backstreet abortions during the 1950s, another compelling reason for Sanger's continued angst over reliable birth control. Even in her senior years, she longed for a better way. She found it quite by accident.

SANGER AND EUGENICS

In the 1920s, Sanger became involved with the eugenics movement, arguing that birth control was especially necessary for the poor, handicapped, and "minorities." Her reasoning rankled many, and put her on the historical record as a bigoted extremist. She wanted easy access to birth control for blacks, immigrants, and the handicapped because they were "human weeds," "reckless breeders," "spawning . . . human beings who never should have been born." Sanger felt that birth control was an important tool in building a strong and vital society: "More children from the fit, less from the unfit—that is the chief aim of birth control." Although some of her comments were outrageous, in historical context, she was in the forefront of a vital women's movement, someone who braved the mean streets of New York's toughest and cruelest neighborhoods. She had done her best to bring the plight of poor and immigrant women, dying from botched abortions and self-inflicted cures for unwanted pregnancy, to the public's attention.

In casual conversation at a dinner party, Sanger aired her complaints to a young biologist named Gregory Pincus. She lamented the lack of safe and reliable birth control for women, especially for poor and minority women, and those with physical or mental limitations. Sanger remained convinced that somehow, somewhere, there must be a way to create a magic little pill that would put birth control in the hands of women and make it safe and effective at the same time. She was ecstatic when Pincus told her that he believed there was a possibility that women's hormones could actually be chemically manipulated in order to prevent conception: that was all the still-feisty feminist needed!

ALMOST THE LAST GASP FOR THE MINI-COMSTOCKS

In spite of the fact that the vast majority of American doctors approved of birth control for the good of families and women's health, anti–birth control laws remained in a number of states. It was a felony in Massachusetts to "exhibit, sell, prescribe, provide, or give out information" about them, and in neighboring Connecticut, it was a crime for a couple to use contraception.

In 1961 Dr. Lee Buxton, chairman of the Yale Medical School Department of Obstetrics and Gynecology, and Estelle Griswold, the executive director of Connecticut Planned Parenthood, got together to challenge those laws. They opened four Planned Parenthood clinics in Connecticut and were promptly arrested for their efforts. By 1965 the pair had taken their case all the way to the Supreme Court, where the old Comstock leftover was shot down as a violation of personal privacy, finally ending a painful era in the history of human sexuality.

Although the story of the early years of pill "R and D" is a complicated one, the bottom line was that the dinner conversation between history's most determined birth control advocate and a little-known scientist led to the most important scientific inquiry—and result—in the history of human reproduction.

The pill's early years were reminiscent of the history of the condom: it, too, inspired many of the same arguments about the morality of birth control, as well as some new ones, like: using drugs to manipulate women's bodies was unnatural, akin to playing God; to be able to pop a pill and voilà, protection, made it too easy for the unmarried to get away with having sex *without consequences*; and even a very angry response from NAACP groups who accused the Planned Parenthood organization and its clinics of providing birth control pills in order to intentionally limit black birthrates.

And the pope weighed in—again.

In 1964 Paul VI, often called one of history's more progressive popes, was making an effort to modernize the Church and its policies. Perhaps surprisingly, by the Church's own count there were many clergymen—at least 75 percent—who embraced the the pill, believing it to be an excellent method of birth control. But through its papal Commission of Population, the Family and Natality, fondly dubbed the Birth Control Commission, the Church stubbornly refused to recognize any kind of birth control for married couples except the "rhythm method," otherwise known as "Catholic" or "Vatican roulette." That was it.

Papal edicts or not though, a significant percentage of Catholic women embraced the pill: usage grew from approximately 25 percent of American Catholics at the time the Birth Control Commission was meeting, to 80 percent by 1980.

The pill also had its ups and downs with the FDA; in 1966, the same year Margaret Sanger died, the industry had its wings clipped—briefly—when the government agency told companies like Searle that they would have to commit to longer-term studies for the new varieties being developed than had previously been required. Side effects had become an issue. But this did not slow down sales or research. In fact, the pill was so popular that President Eisenhower was asked at a press conference whether or not the federal government would be supporting birth control research. His embarrassed reply was that it "is not a proper political or government activity or function or responsibility" and it is "not our business."

Only a few years later, however, in his State of the Union Address of January 4, 1965, President Lyndon B. Johnson cautiously announced his plans to promote the use of birth control—abroad. "I will seek new ways," he told Congress, "to use our knowledge to help deal with the explosion in world population and the growing scarcity in world resources." This statement of support for birth control was not a bold one, but it was the first ever by a sitting president. Johnson was sure that by merely alluding to federal financing of contraception, he might anger Catholic voters across the country: he was not to know just how many Catholic women were already quietly on the pill.

By the mid-1970s, domestically the federal government was helping to fund more than two thousand public health clinics, all of which provided

> ## PINCUS AND THE PILL
> *Gregory Pincus died in his forties of a rare disease caused by the chemicals he experimented with in his lab, many of which had led to the creation of the Pill. His life and death is reminiscent of that of the father of the modern condom; just as men do not don a fallopio before having sex, women do not pop a Pincus. His incredibly important contribution to the modernization of birth control has not really been celebrated.*

A PRESIDENTIAL CHANGE OF HEART
From the **New York Times,** *December 9, 1966:*

The Federal Government has executed a crisp about-face on birth control. Until two years ago, Washington hewed to Dwight Eisenhower's blunt 1959 decree on the issue: but Ike, who has been honorary co-chairman (with Harry Truman) of a private group called Planned Parenthood-World Population for the past two years, has had a change of heart. Only last week, he declared he would "personally support all programs, public or private," that offer birth-control information to families.

poor women with the pill. As other countries adopted its use, by the mid-1980s, more than 80 percent of the world's sexually active women under fifty years of age had taken birth control pills.

HOW ABOUT THAT SEXUAL REVOLUTION?

From the time that the Beatles made their debut in America and the plans were being made to put a man on the moon, the growing movement toward a lasting change in regard to the Western world's sexual mores eclipsed into a remarkable period of extreme sexual liberation, most spectacular among white urban and middle-class youth. Miniskirts, love beads, tie dye, and rock and roll became icons for a new and provocative attitude toward sex. Cities like San Francisco, Amsterdam, New York, and London became city centers for a generation dedicated to "free love," ushering in a period of open sexuality even the ancient Greeks would have been proud of.

This heady mix of the pill and free love has led to the historical dismissal of the condom as an anachronism by the sixties. "Sales dropped. The End" has been the standard footnote. But that casual disregard of a device that had been in use for thousands of years could not be further from the truth. Because though the pill greatly enhanced the new found sexual freedoms of the younger generation, the good old standby did not just go away.

Some months after the pill made its public debut in 1960, condom sales did begin to feel the impact. But it was certainly not a "dead letter." True to its long and tumultuous history, it found its way into the public eye in a number of interesting places throughout the sixties and into the seventies. Just before the "British invasion" of America—which turned the postwar "England copies the United States" trend around—Beatle Paul McCartney made the news when he was arrested in Hamburg, Germany, during an early Beatles tour. He had hung up a condom in a public place and literally set fire to it. Paul thought it was funny, but the German police did not agree, inviting him to leave the country.

> ## YELLOW SUBMARINE
> *Years later, the apparently condom-conscious Beatles made the news again when John Lennon used one to cover his microphone while recording "Yellow Submarine." He liked the sound effect.*

In popular fiction and film, the smash English novel (and later a TV show) *A Kind of Loving* featured Victor embarrassed to be discovered buying a "packet of three" (still the magic number in packaging); as late as 1971, a condom loomed large in the movie *Carnal Knowledge*. Then, the seamy side of Theresa's character emerged in *Looking for Mr. Goodbar* when she let the faceless man she'd just picked up know just what she thought of his suggestion that they practice safe sex—instead of being grateful for the precaution, she blew up the proffered condom before handing it back. In *Steps*, Jerzy Kosinski's dark fiction about the Soviet Union, the author used the condom to help his tortured narrator heap silent scorn on the communist system by having him pin condoms on the chests of hated *apparatchiks*.

But through all this, what was the rubber's role during the sexual revolution?

✦✦✦✦✦

Between 1955 and 1965 approximately 42 percent of Americans of reproductive age used condoms as birth control: it is only within the Jewish and African American communities that usage had dropped by just under 10 percent by 1965. The pill did not challenge these numbers until the 1970s, and then only briefly.

In the United Kingdom, the story is similar; between the years 1950 and

SHE'S TOO MUCH OF A LADY

In dozens of interviews conducted by sociologists in England and the United States, the majority of older married women tut-tutted not at the questions about having sex but at those about their knowledge and use of the condom as birth control. They inferred that that was a "man's business." Queries of older British couples about how they avoided pregnancy in their younger days prompted responses like: "Oh, well, we used, we used to use the, er, French letters we used to call 'em. I don't know, what's the official thing called, what was the expression? Sheaths. The sheath, that's right. Yes, it was the man's option to prevent the children but er . . . it was the man's job."

When asked how they knew about sheaths and where they purchased them, responses were vague, yet enlightening, as they reflected the continued lack of official knowledge about birth control: "Oh, er, you'd find somebody selling them on the corner of the street, or, er, a chemist, chemists mostly, but that's where you learnt about 'em was on a corner of the street, nothing to tell about 'em, only that they were rubber goods, that's all."

Another study on the birth control choices of couples from the 1920s to the 1950s, conducted throughout England in 1960, concluded that as those decades proceeded, British men were increasingly expected to take precautions. The authors of the study concluded with "contraception is still part of the husband's prerogative." This fits other evidence regarding the new birth control clinics opening up on both sides of the Atlantic; women more often than not sought help based on urgings from their husbands, who usually ended up sticking with their French letters, partly out of the comfort of the known and partly because choices at the time were still very limited.

1960, 60 percent of married Britons preferred "male methods of contraception"—sheaths. The pill had outstripped the condom by 1970—from 1966 to 1970, 38 percent of married couples and sexually active singles used the pill, versus 31 percent using the condom—but perhaps somewhat surprisingly, single women still preferred that men take the initiative. This jives with the statistical information from pharmaceutical sales, which showed a much greater comfort zone among women when it came to buying condoms. Interestingly, American women also proved themselves to be more comfortable than men when it came to picking up a packet of Trojans.

The solid status of the condom as first then second choice is perhaps even more intriguing given the state of advertising by the end of the 1950s: American television and radio were officially banned from advertising condoms (or any other form of birth control) by the National Association of Broadcasters (NAB). The ban remained in place throughout the 1970s.

The first commercial to buck that prohibition was aired in California, where in 1975 a Trojan commercial was shown on KNTV. Viewers overwhelmingly approved of the ad, but the station did not like the national attention it drew and yanked it despite its popularity.

This weird media netherworld was reflected in an article titled "In the Shadows," printed in a 1963 edition of *Time* magazine's business section. In the words of the unknown author, "In the ranks of US business thrives a shadow industry, whose presence is largely ignored by businessmen and talked about only discreetly by its managers." *Time* told its readers that though the contraceptive industry was more or less underground, it was growing at an astounding rate, with domestic condom sales going past the $85 million mark that year. The figure is not correct—sales remained steady at about $200 million a year in spite of the pill—but it does reflect a certain ignorance or possibly just naiveté on the part of the media, since there was nothing particularly underground about the sale of condoms at the time, nor was it an up-and-coming industry, but rather one that had been at the pinnacle of Wall Street for many years.

> ## JAPANESE CONDOMS
> In the 1960s, the Japanese used more condoms per capita per year than any other nation, and relied on them as their number one birth control device. As stated by an executive at Okamoto, still Japan's leading manufacturer, "Japanese rely on physical measures rather than chemical measures for contraception." At the same time, they also pioneered a much more comfortable variety, leading the Japanese consumer to reject all condoms made in America or Europe. Their *kondomus* were one one-thousandth of an inch in thickness, half that of foreign brands, and were "favored for their extreme comfort." And, by the 1980s, they were sold door-to-door by a sales force of middle-aged women who worked for the manufacturers.

Perhaps the most, or only, accurate part of the article was its assertion that manufacturers were counting on an increase in sales, figuring that they had tapped only 20 percent of the potential birth control market. They were sure that with the huge wave of baby boom teens now coming of age, there was no where to go but up.

That hope for increased market share was realized beginning in 1967,

INDIAN HOW-TO'S

Packets of condoms were displayed in shop windows, on peddlers' trolleys, even alongside the ducks and chickens strung up in the windows of local butchers. The name chosen for the Indian-made condoms, Nirodh, is Sanskrit for "freedom from fear" and was supposed to help sell the concept and make Indian men willing to spend twenty cents each. But education on just how to use the device was a bit more problematic. Most AID personnel felt that the shape and size of condoms made it obvious how they "worked," while others insisted upon written instructions. Both approaches turned out to be somewhat iffy, so local village elders were employed to demonstrate how to put on a condom. For this they used lengths of bamboo; the problem was when village men placed their condoms over their own bamboo shoots at home, they found that the magic didn't work for them.

when there was a huge increase in demand. But what neither *Time* nor the manufacturers would have been able to predict was what drove that market surge. Because of the Agency for International Development's (AID) push (with presidential support) toward "the great task of solving the world population crisis," by the midsixties countries like India, through grants from the United States, were buying 50 million condoms a year from the United States and at least 22 million from Japanese manufacturers. (By 1970, India was also producing more than 270 million a year.) This new and seemingly endless market opened up quite suddenly when the AID reversed earlier hands-off policies governing birth control and international aid. In fact, American officials were so determined to get Indian men to wear them, that as one AID officer put it, "We want the condom to be as well advertised as Coca-Cola." This was just the beginning of a many-decade push to offer billions of freely distributed *Nirodhs* throughout the third world.

POSTWAR EUROPE—WHAT HAPPENED TO THE GUMMIS?

Like previous eras, after the war those countries that had once been the centers of condom commerce saw a flip-flop in not only usage but sexual mores—and the laws codifying them. Like the pro-birth movement in

France after World War I, fears of a shrinking population once again led many to believe that condoms were a danger to the very existence of France. The pro-natalist movement was back, but this time it proved to be much more powerful than before.

Similar to the extreme feminization of women's roles in the United States and the United Kingdom, French women were expected to go home and stay there, helping to fulfill General de Gaulle's 1945 demand of women to have "en dix ans, douze millions de beaux bébés pour la France" ("twelve million bouncing babies for France in the space of ten years), or "le baby boom." Abortion was a crime punishable by death and birth control was illegal, a fact that did not change until 1967. As with other extreme movements, there were those who chose to ignore the bans, obtaining foreign-made condoms through the black market, but it did make life very difficult for many French couples who simply could not afford too many mouths to feed in an economy racked by war.

The picture was somewhat different in Italy, where, in spite of the looming presence of the Church, there was a very active and public birth control movement that began in the midfifties: in 1956, the Italian Association for Demographic Education (AIED) was founded with the aim of defending the idea and the practice of limiting the number of children a couple decided to have and specifically of combating the existing legislation against birth control. The AIED had an interesting collection of supporters, all secular, including the socialists and the communists, but its proposals were strongly opposed by the Catholics, who outnumbered the others and managed to uphold all anti-condom legislation. Although the laws against birth control remained on the books until 1971 when they were declared unconstitutional, condom use was quite common by the end of the sixties (and had been quietly practiced long before then) and even abortion became legal and easily available during that decade, in spite of the Church's loud and very public opposition.

Perhaps surprisingly, it is in Germany where the gummi and birth control in general suffered the greatest suppression after the war. Hitler's strange notions about human sexuality, as it turned out, had left quite a mark on that country.

The new German republic's government seemed determined in the 1950s to legislate all that it regarded as relating to public and private morality. Although the immediate period after the war was dubbed a time of extreme "erotic liberality," that soon changed: censorship became the norm, and any kind of dissemination of birth control information was strictly prohibited. Like the early Nazi era, access to condoms, in spite of protests, was not completely cut off, though there were those who tried hard to prevent their sales. Just as in the war years, fear of disease, or the handy exploitation of that fear, had kept them on the market, but while vending machines had been fairly common on many German streetscapes, as well as in public toilets and at the backs of bars and barbershops, from the mid-1950s to the early 1960s there were heated debates among jurists and journalists over the desirability of these machines. The argument against them was that even the neutral display of condoms in vending machines could be interpreted, and some courts did, as an offense to "sitte und anstand"—morals and decency.

This vague but effective traditional legal category was often employed by conservative jurists in their efforts to deter youth (and by default, adult) access to birth control. And, like in Italy, Catholic activists set the terms of the conversation; in 1951 and 1952 conservative Catholic youth organizations burned down kiosks that marketed pornography, and in 1953 they initiated actions against condom vending machines. Far from being legally censured, this inspired more street activism—or more accurately, rioting—against condom machines. As the decade progressed, it is not surprising that fewer and fewer young Germans knew much about the private matter of sex and specifically of birth control, ushering in another era of sexual confusion and ambivalence. But then came along Germany's answer to Margaret Sanger.

During World War II, Captain Beate Uhse was the only female pilot in the Luftwaffe; her husband, also a pilot, was killed in action in 1944, leaving her with a baby to raise and a shaky career as a pilot on the losing side. But it was her skill as a pilot that probably saved her and her son's life when she commandeered a plane and flew them out of Berlin just ahead of advancing

Russian forces. She ended up in England, where she was briefly imprisoned, and then allowed to return to Germany a few years later. Upon her arrival home, Beate was stunned to see the unhappy returned soldiers and their wives with no access to birth con-

> ## NO COLD WAR FOR THE CONDOM
> *In spite of the huge changes that had taken place during and after the war, in some ways the Soviet Union and its satellite states were ahead of the Europeans, at least in their straightforward approach to birth control. Condoms were always in demand, and the biggest complaint of Russians was that supply never caught up with demand. Even in little Czechoslovakia, a company with its origins in late nineteenth-century Germany managed to come back in a big way: the VULKAN company did a land office business in natural rubber condoms, and by the 1960s proudly marketed its Primero brand, which was still on Eastern European pharmacy shelves until 2005.*

trol, no money, and too many children to care for. The sexually regressive politics of the times were too much for her and she was determined to do something about it.

Beate, whose mother had been one of Germany's first women doctors and had taught her daughter a great deal about birth control even though such knowledge was not allowed during the Nazi regime, challenged not only the social norms of the time but also the law. She made a quiet deal with a rubber manufacturer and sold the condoms he made for her, along with birth control advice booklets she wrote herself, door-to-door; later, she began a mail-order business selling not only condoms and birth control advice, but sex toys as well. Years later Beate was one of Germany's greatest sex entrepreneurs, in spite of years of legal battles she had had to fight, and with only one exception, she had always won.

By the 1990s, the former pilot owned a chain of popular sex shops whose shares sold well on the German Stock Exchange. When she died, she was not only worth the equivalent of almost two hundred million dollars, Beate was also a highly respected social activist and businesswoman. She was remembered fondly not only as a condom entrepreneur but as the person who brought the once-taboo subject of human sexuality back into the limelight: "Sex, like eating and drinking, is one of mankind's basic needs."

WHAT ABOUT PRACTICAL PROPHYLAXIS?

By 1950, to the tune of two hundred million dollars' worth a year, America's number one choice for birth control was the condom. But before the end of the 1950s, their use as disease preventative had all but gone away. Penicillin and other modern drug therapies had put to rest many age-old health concerns, not the least of which was the dreaded scourge of syphilis. It was also a period when prostitution was at an all-time low in most Western countries. Many historians believe this was due to the postwar drop in the average age of marriage and the quiet but steady lifting of the taboos against premarital sex. Either way, it seemed that fewer prostitutes meant less disease. But this is also a strange time in history in regard to sexual mores, attitudes, and the public versus private approach to sex. Again.

Because of federal government efforts to end VD once and for all, by 1948 there were only seventy thousand Americans afflicted with a sexually transmitted disease, which was actually a remarkable feat given that just the American military alone had reported almost four hundred thousand cases in 1919. By 1957 the eradication effort had been so successful that there were fewer than seven thousand reported cases that year.

Reminiscent of the arguments against the use of condoms and later the pill, there were government officials and doctors who believed that the stunning success of the public education efforts and wonder drugs that had helped make this drop possible was likely to lead to extreme promiscuity and the eventual demise of the family—and society with it—but the success was lauded by most, and by the end of the fifties, the once-abundant funding for clinics and VD eradication programs had all but dried up: after all, syphilis was a thing of the past, right? Sadly, not quite.

> *That's what usually happens. . . . When a disease control program reaches the point of near eradication, it's usually the program that's eradicated, not the disease.*
> Dr. William Holder of the Mississippi Health Department

Even though it appeared that venereal diseases were near extinction, many US and UK public health officials tried to keep their education programs alive; history had proved how necessary it was to educate about the dangers of unprotected sex and how quickly venereal diseases could bounce back. But their message was drowned out by those who now found that message outmoded and downright unsavory. This was, after all, a time when there were few cases on record, early marriage and monogamy were the cultural ideal, and when all else failed, drugs could cure all. Public will and willingness to spend tax dollars on prevention simply dried up.

Then along came the Sexual Revolution.

In the United States and the United Kingdom, family planning clinics, most of which received extensive public funding, were becoming increasingly common and very public about sex education and providing condoms—for birth control. There was no suggestion that VD and birth control clinics be fused, combining both messages and getting the most mileage out of public money—and condoms. Instead, by the early sixties VD eradication programs had all but gone the way of the poodle skirt, and the shrinking educational effort was confined to the quietly growing number of free, privately funded clinics (which were fast becoming a necessity) and underfunded local health departments, where small staffs labored to deal with an exploding yet silent epidemic of venereal disease. And by the time an infected person ended up in one of these facilities, curing—not preventing—was the message.

The not-so-long-term effect was absolute ignorance about the dangers of unprotected sex with the wrong partner. Practical prophylaxis was not even a distant memory for most, especially among the younger generation, which resulted in a

VD TESTING

Wasserman testing became a requirement in order to receive a marriage license in most states at the end of the 1950s. Officials were convinced that this would be a very important step in eradicating VD, and the cases reported by the state's licensing bureaus were those used to report disease incidence in the United States. This explains why so many cases went uncounted and why bean counters were content to slash funding for educational efforts. Total reliance on one test, and one population—the soon-to-be-married—left out the most at-risk populations: poor blacks, urban youth, and the rural poor all suffered because they went uncounted.

venereal plague that rivaled anything the world had ever seen.

"THE AGE OF . . ." VD

By 1965 it was estimated that at least 650,000 Americans under twenty were contracting either syphilis or gonorrhea annually. Estimates for the over-twenties varied, but the numbers were staggering. By 1969 states like Texas, Virginia, Nevada, Illinois, and Tennessee were reporting well over 300 people per 100,000 residents had gonorrhea—Georgia reported more than 500.

Big cities were the hardest hit: Atlanta reported over 2,300 cases per 100,000, and the numbers in Los Angeles, San Francisco, Washington, DC, and Newark were not much better. In Los Angeles alone, officials were sure that over 45,000 women had the disease and did not realize it. That year there were a total of just under 450,000 cases of gonorrhea reported in the United States, and the number of unreported cases was probably much higher. In the case of syphilis, the numbers were not as bad, but it certainly had not gone away. It was similar in the United Kingdom, where the National Health Services increasingly found it difficult to keep up with a burgeoning number of new cases of not only syphilis and gonorrhea but also what came to be known as the "second generation" of sexually transmitted diseases. And in the age of the feminist movement, women, for the first time in history, were as likely to be infected as men.

FROM VD TO STD

Many people think that the phrase "sexually transmitted disease" is a very recent one, but it was actually coined in 1910 by one of the Western world's most important doctors, Sir William Osler. He felt venereal disease was associated only with gonorrhea and syphilis, and wanted something that encompassed the other types of infection that were related to sexual contact. Osler, who was born in Canada but served in important posts at both Johns Hopkins and Oxford medical schools, was in the forefront of the movement to modernize and professionalize medicine and was not shy about pushing to take STD treatment out of the hands of general practitioners, creating a new specialty in the field of medicine. It was, in fact, the British National Health Services that pioneered this idea during the pandemic of the 1960s, though Osler's "new" reference was not officially adopted in the United Kingdom by the Medical Society for Venereal Diseases until 1973.

A doctor who specialized in treating VD summed it all up when he said that "the bugs aren't half as resistant to the drugs as patients are to instruction on prevention." Once again, history was to repeat itself, and nowhere did the mistakes of the past visit themselves more obviously than in the American military.

BACK TO MORAL PROPHYLAXIS

After World War II, the American military, which though slow to catch on, had had a profound effect on bringing the condom into the disease-prevention fold, turned wholeheartedly to character education, with the army experimenting on young recruits by requiring they attend classes on morality and religious instruction. Riveting lectures with titles like "The Ten Commandments," "Purity in Thought, Word, and Deed," and "Marriage as a Sacred Institution" were delivered by chaplains across the country. Gone was the practical "boys will be boys" message that it was better to be safe than sorry. Though the most extreme religious messages never became an army-wide requirement for all recruits, it was the model that influenced certain elements of military training all the way through the Vietnam War, with military officials again trying to make "it" all about the individual soldier's morality—or lack thereof. Sex outside of marriage once again became an issue of misconduct, a punishable offense. And once again, policy did not reflect practice.

During and after the Korean War, a rich army in a poor nation meant there were Korean prostitutes on every corner and the VD rate among soldiers hit historic highs: eight out of ten contracted gonorrhea at least once during a twelve-month stint. Thanks to the "wink-wink-

> ## THAT SOLDIER'S DUMBEST MOMENT
> *That same soldier's dumbest army moment "came on the troop transport to Korea in December, when the afternoon movie one day was the latest Martin & Lewis; the preceding short subject [film] was a WW2 army training film: 'How to take a shower and get a short arm inspection.' With real live models. There was only the sound of mass exodus, a herd of young studs thundering out the exit to the main deck. We all missed that Martin & Lewis film."*

AN KHE PLAZA OR DISNEYLAND EAST

A painful example of the often-bizarre results of war and especially the military's response to "handling" soldier's sexuality is the village of An Khe, a once-sleepy little village in the Central Highlands of Vietnam. When a massive American encampment landed there with twenty-one thousand troops, prostitutes and pimps were right behind them, changing the face of the village and endangering the troops' health; 30 percent of the soldiers contracted VD within the first few weeks of arrival. The commanding officer's response was to allow the village elders to build a brothel whose prostitutes, or "Tea Girls," were handpicked and checked by American doctors, then given high doses of anti-VD drugs. The soldiers referred to this twenty-five-acre "plaza," complete with surrounding barbed wire, as Disneyland. The locals called its many bars and back rooms "boom boom parlors." Either way, though the girls were monitored regularly, condoms also played a conspicuous role in preventing disease and were available at the entrance to every parlor, as well as in the men's rooms.

MILITARY MUZZLES

When things heated up in Iraq, catalog condom sales to soldiers at military bases went up 900 percent. The Pentagon preferred not to comment on the explosion of sales, but when pushed, they responded with vague references to military use of the little items as possible protection from sandy conditions for their weapons. After all, there would be no fraternization between American troops and local women. Sales directors disagreed with the latter, saying that most military men did not like their government-supplied pros, and those were being used to "cover soldier's muzzles."

nod-nod" approach to prevention, there were still pros available, but like the general populace, many men were much less aware of sexual health than their World War II counterparts, and others just figured it was easily cured. This casual attitude meant that in spite of free vending machines—and in the case of the navy and merchant marine, large barrels on the gang plank overflowing with condoms so that sailors could grab a handful every time they went ashore—disease was a given for the average American soldier serving in Korea. It remains a problem there today.

The reality was that there was plenty of affordable sex for sale. Clumsy attempts at education were part and parcel of individual leaders' attempts to be practical, but there was no military-wide program to help support the effort. Some commanding officers actually worked with troops as they headed off to Korea to inform their men about safe sex and the dangers they would face if they were sloppy about protection, but it was too little and often too late. The memory of one soldier's experience of "sex ed in the field" probably sums up the quality of the instruction: "The whole company lined up one snowy morning with our hapless, trying-to-be-serious Top Sergeant standing before us ... with a broomstick stuck through his legs to an appropriate length and at an appropriate angle demonstrating how to apply a condom. True. It was the Second Dumbest Army Moment in my career."

Dumb or not, condoms did help lower the VD rate where crude training was conducted, but as the numbers continued to soar during and after the conflict, throughout the sixties and into the seventies, official support of any such training efforts remained conspicuously absent.

During the Vietnam War, the same problem persisted. One officer complained that "it runs wild out there," referring to the hot and cold running prostitutes. This high-ranking official added that "suppression is our policy. If we can do it suppression is best. Unfortunately, in some areas we just can't do it. . . . We have enough trouble regulating haircuts let alone their sex habits." The pros were available, the education was not.

COMBATING THE PLAGUE, AGAIN

Oh so true to the long and troubled history of the condom, advertising and public discussion of what by the early 1970s was a venereal disease pandemic demonstrates the moral, legal, and ethical struggles inherent in dealing with just how, when, where, to whom (and if) the message of safe sex and protection should be projected. In this, radio and television continued to be conspicuously absent, which is true even today.

In 1977 the puritanical leaders of the NAB met in San Diego to establish a committee to work with TV officials on what those leaders termed an effort "to discuss what additional contributions broadcasters can make in addressing such important national health problems as unwanted pregnancies and venereal disease." As the *New York Times* put it, "That's their way of saying they will discuss broadcast advertising for condoms." But it was not a very serious discussion, given that even by 1979 when the Justice Department had fought and won a battle to overturn the NAB's anticondom code, the change did little to encourage other broadcast media to begin advertising prophylaxis, in spite of the relaxed social-sexual atmosphere left by the sexy sixties.

It is perhaps telling that in a media environment in which one would surely expect to find this kind of advertising, it was actually limited to written publications, mostly men's magazines like *Penthouse*; when Julius Schmid's company had approached *Playboy* in the midsixties with ideas for low-key promotion of its product as birth control in that popular magazine, even its editors refused any mention of condoms because they did not want to "disturb the euphoria of its male readership." To its credit, by the end of the sixties, *Playboy* had turned around its anticondom advertising policy and begun accepting

ADVERTS

Although the English were not so squeamish when it came to condom advertising, birth control was the message the London Rubber Company pushed when it began its first really big print-advertising campaign in 1969. At the same time, laws regarding the public display of sexually oriented materials in retail outlets were loosened and some pharmacies began to display condom packages on the shelves instead of forcing customers to ask for them. British manufacturers also recognized the importance of advertising to women and pushed brands like the comfortable Gossamer line in popular women's magazines like Loving, The Women's Mirror, Brides, and Setting Up Home.

The government had also tightened up on quality control beginning in 1964, when British Standard-BS3704 was enacted. This required manufacturers to date each package, state materials used in production, and test their products rigorously. Even though there were consistently silly rumors that continued to circulate about the evils of condoms, ranging from the vague idea that there was a little-known law that ten or twelve condoms per hundred were required to be faulty, to the notion that Catholic workers in rubber-goods factories secretly pricked the tips of sheaths with a pin, the National Birth Control Association put them on its Approved List of reliable products, which also enhanced the condom's standing—but still only as birth control.

Like Americans, though, British adults increasingly looked to the Pill for protection; this, combined with the fact that modern drug therapy had made fear of sexually transmitted diseases a thing of the past, meant that by the end of the 1950s rarely did Britons use condoms for protection of their health.

ads for the major brands, but only as birth control. *Ebony* and a few lesser-known magazines followed suit, but the other media outlets did not. They remained standoffish when it came to advertising condoms for any purpose.

And in spite of the soaring VD rates, until the 1970s, manufacturers continued to pursue advertisements for their products only as birth control; when it came to disease prevention, the good ol' days of pretty mermaids lounging on a package of widows boldly labeled "For Prevention of Disease" were over. No one wanted to demean their products by identifying them with the growing sexual plague.

BUT WHERE THE BIG BOYS LEFT OFF . . .

To their credit, some of the major magazines and newspapers like *Time* magazine and the *New York Times* did an admirable job of attempting to bring public attention to the venereal disease problem. By running serious articles with titles like "VD: A National Emergency," no one could accuse these high-end sources of trying to avoid publicizing the frightening scourge, but the average American remained uncomfortable with the message, or simply did not read the articles. That and just like the bad old days of epidemics gone by, grassroots efforts had proven time and again to be the only way to get the message to everyone. Those efforts would take a lot of time and money to resurrect.

By 1970 there were entrepreneurs, educators, private organizations, nonprofits, and local health departments who recognized that the skyrocketing VD rates had to be addressed. A small not-for-profit called Population Services Inc., run out of a second-floor office in North Carolina by a British doctor, T. R. L. Black, and a former deputy director of CARE, Philip Harvey, a character who would loom large in condom history more than two decades later, exemplified this private effort to address a growing public menace. These men focused their attention on young college students, trying to help them understand just how simple and inexpensive condoms really were in protecting against disease. They advertised in thousands of college publications, so that at least the students of Rutgers and Berkeley—who bought condoms by the gross from PSI's mail-order business, responding to catchy ads like "What will you get her for Christmas . . . pregnant?"—got the dual message of birth control and safe sex, and students in small-town colleges who knew about the catalog ordered their devices in private rather than making the embarrassing trip to the town's local drug store. Retail anonymity meant safer sex. Given the fact that it was still illegal to send condoms through the mail, it was also risky.

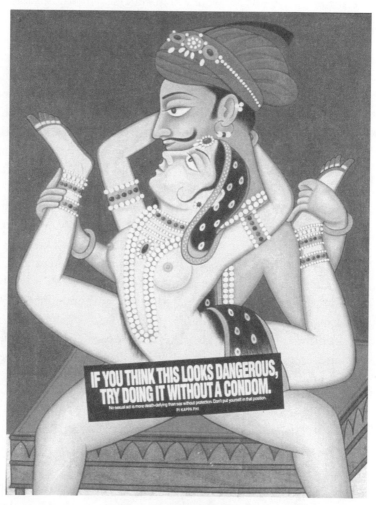

US college poster: the "Kama Sutra"

The old standby "public education," specifically in schools, was still being haggled over by the early seventies, when it was suggested by leading experts that children as young as twelve should be taught the safe-sex message. Some experts believed that a national program for mandatory testing for forty million Americans would help officials end the problem, but that brought up the issue of cost. Public health advocates were doubtful that the national will to spend that much, when gas prices loomed large and the Vietnam War had done so much harm to the national psyche, existed.

In places like Sacramento, California, there were local attempts to promote condom use, while nationally the National Commission on Venereal Disease was busy calling for a study on "research into *prophylaxis* and wide public education on the method." More than fifty years after the military had first been swamped with VD and the message of prevention had percolated through the public and private ranks, and thirty years after the "Put it on before you put it in" motto had saved countless lives and a lot of public monies, it was back to studying up on whether condoms were helpful in preventing venereal disease. And the old argument about "public health officials educating about and supplying condoms was a green light to illicit sex" reared its head again. At a time when government and individuals could afford to retreat into fear and ignorance, it would seem that history would again repeat itself. The supposed open-mindedness of the Age of Aquarius apparently had its limits.

In hopes of finding a blanket solution to the pandemic, in 1972 the commission asked for forty-six million dollars to be spent in the next fiscal year in order to help find the cure to the modern plague. But little did they know that this was only the beginning.

"IF ONLY . . ."

In the "what ifs" of history, it is tempting to consider just how different the world would be in the twenty-first century if what had been known for so many centuries had been embraced as common and consistent practice by the twentieth century. If at some point the condom had finally been accepted as a practical and moral device instead of forever being batted about as some kind of whipping boy for the ups and downs of human sexuality, or the perception of it, perhaps history's worst pandemic might never have happened. Sadly, though, no one could have predicted what the next and most dramatic surge of contagion would mean to the world.

FIFTEEN

abstain was all he said

IN THE AGE OF AIDS

s the seventies moved forward, the world seemed to get smaller and technology was king: Bill Gates founded Microsoft, postal workers worried that they would be replaced by e-mail—Queen Elizabeth II was the first head of state to send one—cell phones were born, and so was the first test-tube baby. American teens went nowhere without their Sony Walkmans.

The movie *Love Story* brought tears to the eyes, while *Ms.* magazine illustrated the new feminism, and Stephen King scared the pants off devoted readers. *Saturday Night Live* satirized American society and *The Godfather* set box office records. Alexander Solzhenitsyn was the first Russian to win the Nobel Prize in Literature and Jamaica exported reggae to the delight of people around the world.

By the eighties, Ronald Reagan reenergized the American presidency, the Berlin wall fell along with the USSR, closing the final chapter of the cold war. The British fought in the Falklands, and privatized many of their national industries. Stephen Hawking brought the study of space down to earth with his *A Brief History of Time*, and *The Simpsons* would go on to be one of the most popular cartoons ever. The whole world saw the brutal nature of Chinese communism, as the Tiananmen Square massacre was broadcast around the world; Salman Rushdie became public enemy number one of the Muslim world with the publication of his *Satanic Verses*, while the Nobel Prize was awarded for the first time to a book written in Arabic. Everyone had a Rubik's Cube and the first woman justice was appointed to the US Supreme Court, while England ushered in a new age when Margaret Thatcher became its first woman prime minister. The Internet was "on," faxing was born, and the laptop became a new computer necessity. In spite of the sixties' call for sensitivity to the natural world, the worst environmental disasters in history turned Bhopal and Chernobyl into dead zones, while the Iran-Contra scandal left America's Teflon president shaken, not stirred.

By 1970 the United States was spending $6,300,000 a year on tracking down the sexual partners of those who had been diagnosed with venereal diseases, and $30,000,000 on VD education. Little money, however, was dedicated to research on prevention, including trying to understand current sexual norms, information the experts on VD desperately needed to fight epidemics. Commitments flip-flopped, as research projects were funded then defunded because of political opposition to the intimate, and some thought, obscene, nature of such research. Others, like two legislators from New York, felt monies spent on that kind of research was pointless: "Never has it been more true than in this situation that an ounce of prevention is worth a pound of cure. The prophylactic is a simple, inexpensive preventative of venereal disease." True, but . . .

> ## SCANDINAVIA'S APPROACH
> Not long after the European VD endemic was publicized, the Scandinavian nations lost no time in following up. Without prudery or false morality, they made sure that condoms were available everywhere and that they were free. The public information campaign was a straightforward, no frills affair—and the Swedes, for instance, suffered almost no contagion at all. That continues to be the case today.

As the seventies wore on, desperate public health officials tried to understand just who were the most at-risk populations, and the findings were disturbing: small, locally funded studies found that though a bare majority of teens polled understood that condoms helped protect against disease, they did not really understand just what STDs could do to their health; most also thought they needed parental consent to obtain condoms, which meant they did not understand that they could buy a *packet of three* in any pharmacy or chain drug store. And, only a minority had any knowledge of how to actually use a condom. The most at-risk teens, African Americans, knew little about protection of any sort, including birth control. Meanwhile, the number of gonorrhea cases continued to soar. In fact, there was another dramatic increase of most STDs, including the appearance of new varieties.

THE NUMBERS GAME

Through the seventies, along with the emergence of penicillin-resistant strains of gonorrhea, syphilis was also on the rise in certain populations. But that is just the beginning. By the 1980s cases of genital herpes were eleven times higher than in the seventies; by 1989 the Centers for Disease Control and Prevention (CDC) found that thirteen million people in the United States were newly infected with one or more symptomatic STDs. Even this was only the tip of the iceberg given that many forms of VD are not noticeable, making it likely that some would go undiagnosed, while others were not on the list of diseases doctors were required to report.

By 1990, 670,000 new cases of gonorrhea were being reported per year in the United States, a number health officials believed to be half of the actual cases. Chlamydia eclipsed that with at least 4 million new cases a year. Syphilis reached its highest level since 1950, with more than 48,000 new cases. The CDC believed that 200,000–500,000 new cases of genital

> ## HPV . . . THE *NEW* EXCUSE
> *Human papillomavirus is actually a family of infections, some of which are spread through casual skin contact, some through sexual-specific contact. HPV can cause cervical cancer. Because it is not always a sex-specific disease, condom critics have used it as an excuse to state that they are not effective against all STDs.*

herpes and a million human papillomavirus (HPV) cases per year were being contracted. Trichomoniasis was also spreading quickly, but as an STD that doctors and health agencies were not required to report, accurate numbers were difficult to obtain; officials did know, however, that by 2000 the human papillomavirus, trichomoniasis, and chlamydia accounted for 88 percent of all new cases of STDs among fifteen- to twenty-four-year-olds. In spite of this, between 1979 and 1988, and again at the end of the 1990s, unprotected sex among this age group continued to rise.

Conversely, by the early 1980s many European nations were experiencing a dramatic decline in gonorrhea, probably because of better case detection, more effective treatments, and public education. This did not mean that STDs were not a problem in other developed nations, but the United States and then the United Kingdom led the way in what appeared to be a never-ending cycle of sexually transmitted infections. Then along came AIDS.

Public health officials around the world had dubbed this the period of the worst sexual plague in history, but venereal diseases were all but forgotten when on June 5, 1981, the CDC issued its first warning about a relatively rare form of pneumonia among a small group of young gay men in Los Angeles.

The era of free love was over, but the never-ending condom controversy was about to go into overdrive.

AN UNLIKELY ADVOCATE?

The *New York Times* published its first news story on AIDS on July 3, 1981. In 1982, the CDC formally established the term Acquired Immune Deficiency Syndrome (AIDS), and reported that the four groups who were susceptible to the new disease were: gays, intravenous drug abusers, Haitians, and hemophiliacs. On October 18 that same year, *ABC World News Tonight* was the first to broadcast a discussion on AIDS, warning that the cause was still unknown, but the disease was spreading across the United States.

MARRIAGE AND MONOGAMY

In his column called "Observer," Russell Baker was referring to then president Ronald Reagan when he said "abstain was all he said." His reflections encapsulated what so many Americans were feeling at the time, and proved that the condom pendulum just kept swinging:

To stop the spread of AIDS President Reagan advises virginity unto the marriage altar and monogamy ever after. That would probably do it, all right, but the President has yet to follow through with advice on how to bring back those two old lifesavers.

I say "bring back" because I have the impression that both were already long gone from the American scene by the time the Puritans made Hester wear the "A."

Lately, of course, you might have got the impression that nobody in years has even heard of virginity and monogamy. This is the consequence of science, which came up with contraceptive pills and penicillin. After that, an entire generation wallowed in a vision of paradise: sex without consequences.

I use the word "wallowed" by design. With the pill to undo fertility, antibiotics to remove the danger of venereal disease and easily available marijuana to give their congress a pickup when regularity and inconsequentiality made it pall, we had the first generation in history able, in Joseph Epstein's fine phrase, to enjoy splendor both in and on the grass.

Now it turns out there are consequences after all: AIDS. The consequence of that is that in family newspapers you are now likely to read the word "condom."

These are bad days indeed. I don't like seeing "condom" in my newspaper any more than President Reagan does, and I don't like having the great TV anchormen of America saying "condom" when the whole family, including Grandmother, is gathered in the parlor for news of the latest murders and bombings.

On the other hand, the idea of AIDS being circulated around town is even more distasteful. In bad days you have to settle for the lesser evil.

President Reagan is trying to wiggle out of this bleak necessity when he says the trick is virginity followed by monogamy. When the health authorities in his Government propose educating American youth in the lifesaving efficacy of condoms his response is a wince, detectable in his suggestion that "abstinence" is the best policy.

There is a distinctly nutty quality in the President talking about abstinence. It is as though he were utterly out of touch with his own world, which is show business.

It was at this time that a rather unlikely character became America's most strident condom spokesperson. Despite the fact that he was chosen by Ronald Reagan as much for his staunch conservatism as for his medical expertise, as surgeon general, Dr. C. Everett Koop pushed hard for public education about prevention.

Although Koop did promote abstinence as the first line of defense against disease, he was a very pragmatic physician who knew that the only practical way to keep sexually active people free from disease was to educate them about condoms. On the other hand, in spite of the fact that President Reagan had nominated Koop, when it came to AIDS and prevention, Reagan remained mute for years, adopting the view that harked back to an earlier time—AIDS was the disease of homosexuals (this in spite of his friendship with actor Rock Hudson, one of the first celebrities to contract it) and illicit drug users. Therefore, they got what they deserved.

"ABSTAIN WAS ALL HE SAID"

AIDS advocates have long asserted that Reagan's lack of leadership significantly hindered research and educational efforts to fight the disease, allowing it to get a foothold first in the United States, then the world. In fact, many believe that the strange "on again, off again" of funding for federal research and initiation of national education about AIDS was due to Reagan's antiquated—homophobic—beliefs. But his surgeon general, who wrote after he had retired that "political meddlers in the White House" had compli-

CELEBRITY AIDS

Even the death of his old friend Rock Hudson did not persuade Reagan to change his mind about AIDS. Other famous victims of the disease include ballet's Rudolf Nureyev, tennis star Arthur Ashe, Olympic champion Greg Louganis, Queen's Freddie Mercury, and basketball great Magic Johnson.

cated his work on the disease, and that "at least a dozen times I pleaded with my critics in the White House to let me have a meeting with President Reagan," showed a remarkable commitment to national health and dragged the country into his campaign despite his boss.

In fact, this conservative US surgeon general worked with the CDC on a brochure intended to educate *all* Americans; in 1988, *Understanding AIDS* was mailed to every US household, and it included a full page of information about condom use. One of the statements made in that document, "Condoms are the best preventative measure against AIDS besides not having sex and practicing safe behavior," became a lightening rod of controversy for the anti-condom movement, which would gain momentum in the late 1990s.

THE FEDERAL GOVERNMENT AND AIDS

Government response blew hot and cold throughout the eighties, with bigots like Jesse Helms struggling to keep the epidemic a "private affair" and Reagan pretending it did not exist. But activists did not give up and continued to fight for increased funding for improved treatment, legal rights, and education for victims and the general public. And, there were rays of hope on the government front. In 1988 the US Health Omnibus Programs Extension (HOPE) Act authorized federal funding of education and testing for AIDS, a move that gained momentum by the 1990s under President Bill Clinton.

HELMS AND THE "SINNER'S DISEASE"

In 1987 North Carolina senator Jesse Helms pushed the Helms Amendment, or the "no promo homo," through the US Congress, which effectively banned the use of federal funds for AIDS education. Helms was famous for his prejudices, including his hatred of those with AIDS. He felt that victims were simply being punished for their sins. With statements like "The only way to stop AIDS is to stop the disgusting and immoral activities that continue to spread the disease," and "There is not one single case of AIDS in this country that cannot be traced in origin to sodomy," he left little doubt about how he felt. In 1990 Helms sealed his reputation as America's most high-visibility homophobe when he offered an amendment to the Hate Crimes Statistics Act, trying to prevent AIDS victims from claiming violent acts committed against them as hate crimes.

His reasoning? "The homosexual movement threatens the strength and survival of the American family."

His solution? "State sodomy laws should be enforced."

AIDS activists response? In 1991 a thirty-five-foot inflated condom was put on the roof of his home.

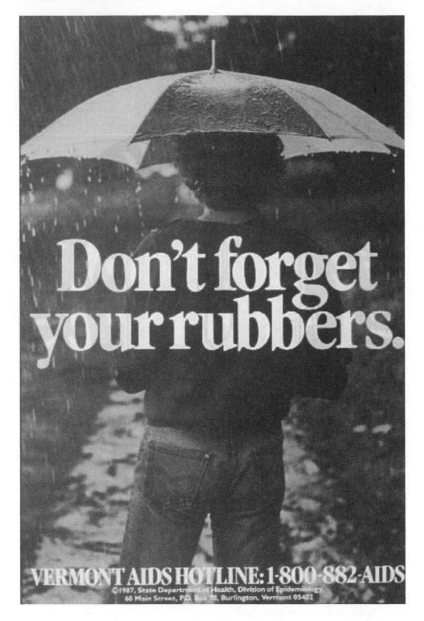

Everybody has a responsibility to get the word out to people that
this product will save lives and prevent a lot of unhappiness.
A condom manufacturer's representative on the need to advertise

Julius Schmid's and Merle Youngs's handsome wartime profits pale in comparison to those of the age of AIDS. At a time where literally anyone could end up with the most mysterious disease since the Black Death, the marketplace was poised to profit, or as John Silverman, president of one of the world's largest manufacturers of condoms, put it: AIDS was "a condom marketer's dream."

The Centers for Disease Control is doing its part with public ser-
vice announcements, manufacturers are doing their part by
making the best possible products, and retailers are doing their
part by fulfilling their responsibility to make the products avail-
able. If we all do our part, we will see growth in the category as
well as doing a great human service.
A condom manufacturer's spokesperson

The giant advertising agency Saatchi and Saatchi apparently agreed since it was one of the first to contribute its considerable marketing skills to an early—and very controversial—series of public service TV, radio, and newspaper announcements for the New York City Department of Health. The straightforward slogans included "Don't go out without your Rubbers," and "Bang. You're Dead! That's how serious AIDS is . . ." were intended to get the attention of those who might otherwise ignore the message. It was perhaps because of the controversy sur-

THE PROBLEM WITH PORN
The largest national market in the 1980s was Japan's, where the condom had been the most popular contraceptive for many years. The Japanese had never embraced the Pill the way Westerners had, preferring their kondomus, to the tune of 68 percent of married couples—864 million condoms each year, three times the unit sales of the United States, whose population was more than twice that of Japan. This fact did not alter significantly until the mid-2000s, when a sharp drop in condom sales was blamed on online porn; more watching, less "doing."

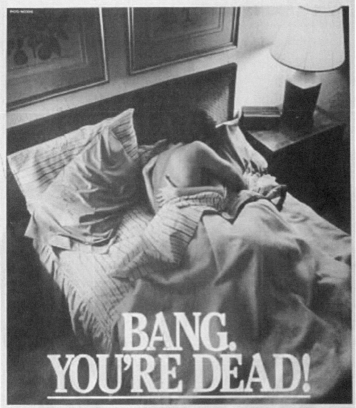

rounding such high-visibility ads that the company chose not to direct them at a wider audience or a very important segment of the population; though AIDS was thought of as a gay disease, the campaign was directed at a heterosexual audience.

Most PSAs used scare tactics and pushed condom use as the only thing between lovers and disease. Although this was an age-old message, to most if not all Americans, the idea was brand new. Consistent with the long history of the humble little condom, things had not changed that much by the late twentieth century.

In spite of the fact that ABC ran a public service announcement about condom use in 1986, and Koop pressured other networks to do the same the following year, only 7 percent aired during prime time, and those were seen during news programming. The rest were broadcast between eleven PM and six AM. Even with the pressure from the surgeon general, the vice president of NBC stated that executives "anguished over these spots quite a while and eventually took the milder ones"; their caution proved timely, because when the few prime-time ads were aired, the networks were inundated with complaints from viewers who were offended by the message. It took more than a decade after the discovery of AIDS—and many decades after the STD epidemic—to get the first commercials, with the exception of that lonely 1975 Trojan ad in California, aired.

In 1991 Fox Television became the first network to air a condom manufacturer's commercial. Yet another decade had to pass before CBS and NBC followed suit; ABC, UPN, and WB all maintained policies against this *type* of

> ## A *NEW YORK TIMES* EDITORIAL: "SEX IS A SERIOUS MATTER"
> The advertisements will not solve all our problems, and invariably some will be offensive. There are commercials as well as programs that are offensive now; they trivialize serious subjects. On the other hand, condom advertisements may do some good, and the risks they present to the social fabric may be worth taking. This critic believes they are. It is just possible the advertisements could save lives. It is also just possible they could help to legitimatize the idea that sex is a serious matter. Thoughtfully done, they would at least be a step toward countering the commercials and programs that relentlessly indicate that sex, practiced only for fun, has no responsibilities attached.
>
> TV View; The Question of Condom Ads
> John Corry, February 8, 1987

advertising. And Fox, though a leader of sorts, banned any ads stating that they were a birth control device. Oh my, how the pendulum had swung.

Further, the industry did not use its potential political capital or its considerable profits to promote its lifesaving product on TV, sticking mostly to the written media and improved methods of packaging and in-store promotion. Individual network affiliates showed a little more daring, as they did choose to air some ads, cherry-picking according to their own demographics.

Radio stations did the same, with individual stations deciding whether or not to carry ads according to their audience. By 1987 one radio station in Indianapolis had carried a Lifestyles ad, but that was a rarity.

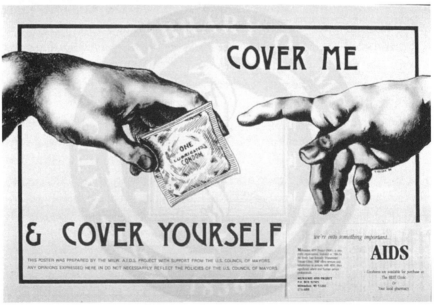

YOUNGS VERSUS TITLE 39

Part of the condom industry's reluctance to advertise in the early days of the AIDS crisis was due to the fact that there were still laws that limited the right to do so.

In 1983 case number 81-1590 was brought to the US Supreme Court. In a move that was painfully reminiscent of the Comstock era and no doubt had Merle Youngs turning over in his grave, the postal service had invoked a section of Title 39 that "prohibits the mailing of unsolicited advertisements for contraceptives" to prevent Youngs Drug Products Corporation from using the mail service to send out educational pamphlets. The company had planned to send the information to targeted areas around the United States; these contained information about AIDS, other STDs, and methods of prevention, including condom use. True to its founder's philosophy, the company chose to fight the ban, claiming it violated the First Amendment. The court agreed. That did not, however, spur the rest of the industry to attempt any like-uses of the mail to get the message of prevention out to everyone.

KOOP'S NUMBERS

Surgeon General Koop urged PSAs be aimed at the most at-risk groups, emphasizing the need to reach blacks and Hispanics. Although Hispanics made up only 6 percent of the population at that time, they made up 14 percent of AIDS victims; blacks, who were 12 percent of the population, accounted for 25 percent. Even by the late nineties, advertising—public and commercial—did not reflect those numbers, however. And, even though women were the latest victims, with the number of female victims equaling and in some places, outstripping those of men, by 2000 only 30 percent of ads featured women. Of those, most had the woman leaving the decision to use protection—or not—up to the man.

SCARY VERSUS FUNNY

I'll do a lot for love, but I'm not ready to die for it . . .
A Lifestyles condom ad

The first wave of commercials about AIDS and condom use carried distinctly scary messages, playing up and on fear. There were some with highly emotional vignettes like the one featuring a young Hispanic man recalling how he had warned his brother that if he was going to have sex, he needed to use a condom, but the brother had replied: "Condoms aren't macho." The boy then knelt down, leaned over his brother's grave, and cried, "My brother. He was so macho."

> *What is disappointing to us is the category is not growing as much*
> *as it should. So much of our target audience is young people who*
> *either don't think they are going to get AIDS, or by the time they*
> *do get it, think there will be a cure for it.*
>
> A statement by a condom industry spokesperson

PRODUCT, PRICE, PROMOTION

By 1994 scary gave way to much lighter fare, where humor became the primary method of getting the safer-sex message across. Some critics went so
far as to call the new ads "vaudevillian" as they featured the Phantom of the
Opera sweeping into a pharmacy to buy his *packet*, only to be told by the
clerk that he did not need a mask to buy condoms; another with Robin
Hood doing the same, except that he winked and informed the cashier the
packs were for him and "for all my merry men." And so the new ads went,
with a cast of outrageous characters assuring the viewer it was great fun to
buy, and therefore use, protection.

The reason for the dramatic turnabout in approach was because, by
1994, condom sales were flat for the first time since before the discovery of
AIDS; industry leaders realized that scare tactics were no longer working
and were desperate to find a new way to deliver an old message. The drop
in sales—and use—was blamed on the notion that although at least
220,000 people had died of AIDS by that year, other issues had captured
the public's attention. The media, and therefore its audience, was distracted

THE FIRST MR. BUSH AND THE AIRING OF "FILTH"

In 1991 George Bush was displeased with the news, what with a Kennedy rape trial, Anita
Hill's sexual harassment charges against Supreme Court nominee Clarence Thomas, and Magic
Johnson's revelation about having HIV. He complained about the "filth and indecent material"
that Americans were exposed to on television and radio. About AIDS, Bush criticized programs
trying to combat the disease by giving condoms to teenagers: "This is a disease that can be
controlled for the most part by individual behavior. I don't think passing out condoms is the
way you affect individual behavior. I don't think that just passing out condoms, giving up on
lifestyle and giving up on family and fundamental values is correct."

by Bosnia, Whitewater, and other national and international news; AIDS took a backseat. That, and "message fatigue" had set in. Top sellers spent millions and millions of dollars on campaigns designed by some of the best advertising firms in the country in an attempt to turn that around.

Niche marketing was also a very important new strategy, with women, minorities, and teens being the focus of campaigns speaking just to those groups. Even in the 1980s, the majority of condoms were still sold through traditionally acceptable retail outlets, the drug stores, but by the nineties, Wal-Mart, Target, and K-Mart were offering a variety of brands, with supermarkets following suit.

Besides the expanded venues, the industry also recognized that a simple sales strategy was to place them not just with the pharmaceuticals, but with soaps, feminine products, and vitamins. Now shoppers could toss a pack of Ramses into the same cart with the milk and bread.

Given that women were the majority spenders in these retail outlets, it made sense to focus on them in some of the ad campaigns and to expand merchandising in women-centric locations, which helped promote a trend begun in the 1980s; women, it turned out, were actually more comfortable buying condoms than men, especially single women. New, more artful packaging, so different from the old-time focus on an all-male market of eighteen- to thirty-four-year-olds, with its macho packaging—like Schmid's Egyptian Ramses and Youngs's helmeted warrior Trojan, associated with vending machines in men's rooms and brown paper packages from "behind the counter" —also gave sales a boost. American women were also realizing—again—that the condom was a reliable birth control method. Although the pill remained the most popular choice for birth control, condoms were a strong second with single women and third choice with married couples.

TIKTOK—EVEN MICKEY D'S GETS INTO THE ACT

By the mid-nineties, McDonald's was feeling the pinch of competition from Burger King and other fast-food restaurants, and corporate leaders were looking for ways to diversify. One such idea was to invest in a new twenty-four-hour mega-vending-machine chain, Tiktok, which offered two hundred products classified as "household necessities," a sort of coin-operated 7-Eleven. The necessities included a variety of condoms, of course.

In recognition of the fact that women by the eighties were buying about 50 percent of the condoms sold by drug stores and other mass retail outlets, Schmid introduced a new brand, Koromex, to appeal just to them; catheter manufacturer Mentor Corporation also entered the "women-only" market.

"COMING OUT OF THE DRAWER"

Although British condoms had been advertised in circulars and handbills for centuries, even with the VD epidemic of the sixties and seventies, by law big companies like Durex could only push their products through print ads; these began in earnest when in 1967 the National Health Services Act allowed public health facilities to begin providing sheaths to unmarried people. Since at that time the company was the only contractor providing them to the NHS, the company decided that monies spent on ads in women's magazines and newspapers like the *Observer* might increase sales to that agency. But the other, more mainstream newspapers and magazines were not interested in that sort of business.

Broadcasting was even more restrictive; though the outright ban on condom advertising on TV had been lifted by the early seventies, companies were not allowed to use their brand names, nor were they allowed to mention disease prevention; the British Code of Advertising Practice demanded commercials "not contain anything deemed offensive to decency." As usual the idea that condoms were a protection against disease had been deemed offensive by television executives for a long time and it took AIDS to change that. The first television and radio advertisements for Durex and Mates were aired in 1987, and they received little public criticism.

In the United Kingdom, the first victim of AIDS was identified in 1981 after he had returned from a trip to the United States; a year later, seven cases had been identified, but it was not until 1983 that British media began to take notice of the disease. Sadly, the initial coverage of the new contagion only served to fuel prejudices against its victims when sensationalist press references to the "Gay Killer Bug" and "March of the Gay Plague" splashed across newspaper headlines. It took another four years for government officials to take the problem seriously.

By 1987 there were 1,170 reported cases of AIDS. In response to the rapid increase, the National Health Services decided to embark on a national campaign titled "Don't Die of Ignorance." The nationwide campaign included a leaflet by that title, which was delivered to every household in the United Kingdom. This was no doubt what influenced American surgeon general C. Everett Koop to do the same the following year. The TV and radio campaigns, featuring icebergs and gravestones, were intended to scare the public into paying attention to the problem and their own sexual health. In a complete turnaround from the days of condoms deemed too obscene for the public airwaves, the national campaign included enlisting major TV presenters to demonstrate on prime time how to use a condom, something that quite a few newspapers reported as distasteful, but government officials received very few complaints from the public; the eighty-million-pound effort was believed to have worked, as the number of AIDS cases leveled off the following year.

MOVE OVER DUREX, GOOD-DAY *MATES*

Before the government sponsored-campaign, Durex was England's only real condom producer, with 95 percent of the market. And then along came Virgin business tycoon–philanthropist Richard Branson.

Branson contributed more than five million pounds of his own money to begin production, with no return to himself, of a new condom brand he called Mates. His unorthodox idea was to sell his new brand through high-visibility retail outlets at no profit to those businesses. A real nonprofit condom.

In order to get Mates off to a roaring start, he also used his considerable clout in the business world to convince some of the world's most famous advertising agencies to come up with a splashy ad campaign—again, at no profit to themselves. As it turned out, the competition was fierce, with agencies recognizing that if they were successful in creating a market for this new condom, they would benefit in a number of ways. First, they would be associated with one of Europe's most high-visibility business interests—Virgin—which could be quite profitable. They would also appear to be the good guys trying to help save the United Kingdom from a growing health crisis. Or as one ad executive put it, "Charity ads are big business."

> *You make love, they make sense.*
>
> Mates advertising slogan

> *Not only do they look great, but they're less expensive, less embarrassing to buy, and Virgin and MTV are going to give all our profits to help stop the spread of sexually transmitted infections.*
>
> Richard Branson

Although there was a lot of backbiting over who would get the account, the final product was much more lighthearted than the government-sponsored campaign, helping to eliminate the stigma that had always accompanied condom advertising. Unlike the somber government approach, the Mates ads attempted to put a humorous slant upon the issue with a teenaged boy entering a pharmacy ready to buy his condoms only to come face to face with a gorgeous woman clerk. In a voice-over, their thoughts are conveyed as the boy tries to screw up the courage to ask for his *packet of three.* It concludes with him courageously asking for a pack and the woman yelling to her boss, "How much for the condoms?!"

Some might have preferred Saatchi and Saatchi's sassier approach, "If it's not on, it's not on," perhaps inspired by the World War II slogan "Remember to put it on before you put it in," but Branson felt that was a bit too risky and opted for something more subtle.

Mates stirred controversy when Branson approached the British Broadcasting Company (BBC), the government-operated noncommercial TV and radio producer, to run his ads on its channels as public service announcements. He offered to have his commercials edited so that the Mates label did not appear, convincing the head of the agency that by trimming out any brand-name reference, he was not getting a freebie, but performing a public good. Durex did not agree, and for the first time in that company's long history, management was fearful that they would lose their

SOCIALIST SHEATHS

Part of the reason London Rubber Company, the makers of Durex, had remained the dominant force in condom production and sales was because of direct government control over pricing, something that had been in place since 1982, but had existed at some level for years. This, along with the fact that the National Health Services represented 23 percent of the market and because the prophylactics they distributed were free, demanded a deeply discounted product—the socialist condom. All these limits meant that newcomers needed a lot of cash up front to enter the business.

overwhelming percentage of the market; faced with the dual prospect of Branson's ten-million-pound ad campaign run on commercial television stations like MTV, and the BBC's gratis public service announcements, it was probably a legitimate fear.

Over Durex's objections, the BBC ran the edited commercials; that same year condom use went up 20 percent in the United Kingdom, encouraging other newcomers to test the market. American, Japanese, and German companies all recognized the potential, and new labels showed up in many retail outlets that not long before had never sold sheaths.

By the end of 1987, Mates—which was manufactured by Ansell—had begun to make real inroads in the English market, including its brand directed at seventeen- to twenty-four-year-olds. Jiffi, whose ad slogans were not meant for a conservative market, offered "Safe-Play" and "Young People's Brand," which came in slick cigarette boxes and proclaimed "Real men do it in a Jiffi," "If she's game and wants your plonker, wear a Jiffi so you can bonk her," and "Only wankers don't use condoms."

In spite of all the hand wringing over loss of market share, Durex did not do too badly out of the newfound interest in their market. To remain competitive, it launched its first-ever promotional campaign, MillionAID, to raise money for charity—and to keep Durex in the public eye. The concept was that for every packet of condoms returned to participating retailers, the London Rubber Company would give ten to twenty pence for each, depending on the size of the pack, up to 250,000 pounds total. The catch was that the boxes had to bare a Kitemark, the government's official stamp telling consumers that that brand had been tested for quality—only Durex and one other label bore that mark in 1987.

NO "GAY" ALLOWED

In spite of the fact that AIDS had been thought of as the "the gay plague" very early on, condom advertising steered clear of using gay themes in their television or radio announcements. In the United Kingdom, the first—for Durex— aired in 1998.

THE BODY SHOPS

Another of England's entrepreneur/philanthropists, Anita Roddick, was one of the few retailers who was more than willing to sell Mates in her cosmetic chain of stores, The Body Shops, at no profit to her company. Others were not so generous, which forced Branson to allow them to sell his brand with a built-in profit margin. Still, between Roddick's Body Shops (and Branson's Virgin record stores) sales at no-profit, and the lower profit margin for those not so willing to do it for free, Mates sold for about ten pence to fifteen pence, versus Durex, which went for about twenty-five pence.

JIFFI QUICK— JUST A HOMONYM?

It is hard to say whether or not the marketer responsible for naming the Jiffi label had a sinister sense of humor as well a very good knowledge of word meanings, but either way, if the average buyer of the brand had any idea about the latter, it might not have sold so well. Jiffy, the correct spelling, is an actual unit of time: one one-hundredth of a second.

In responding to the criticism of the suspect nature of this charitable act, Durex received the backing of the *Daily Mirror*'s own Robert Maxwell, who was then chairman of the National AIDS Trust and apparently sensitive to the coincidental timing of the campaign— hurriedly planned weeks ahead of Branson's own. When questioned about its legitimacy, he stated, "It is commercially right for LRC and it happens to be perfectly right for the public. We need more people to use condoms. I am not an LRC shareholder, I might add." His business dealings, later revealed, may not have made him the ideal spokesperson for the importance of condom use, given it was discovered later that he had stolen over four hundred million pounds from the *Daily Mirror* Trust.

Controversy or no, Durex thrived, acquiring the Italian brand Hatu-Ico the same year, adding another five million pounds a year in sales. It also saw its sales go up over 50 percent, or more than twenty-five million pounds' worth in 1988. But that was just the beginning; in a few years, the once Britain-only company went on to become a powerful global entity.

> ## THAT PESKY OLD PROBLEM
> *By the mid-nineties, the US Food and Drug Adminis-tration found that 20 percent of all condoms tested did not pass the water test—they leaked. The English nonprofit agency Rubberstuffers, which distributed free condoms in gay bars, commissioned the British Standards Institution's laboratories to carry out even more stringent strength tests on a variety of brands sold in the United Kingdom. The results raised some of the same concerns, but also an interesting concern about European Union standards versus the English. The Kitemark was a guarantee of quality only in the United Kingdom, but many consumers there and in Europe believed that the EU's "CE" mark guaranteed the same. It did not, which meant and continues to mean that without one standard of excellence for all of Europe, even so late in the age of AIDS, it con-tinues to be caveat emptor for consumers.*

With the final successes of his campaign to end igno-rance and shame in regard to the purchase and use of con-doms, Branson opted to sell the Mates brand—through his charity the Virgin "Healthcare Foundation"— to the Australian condom producer Ansell Interna-tional, a UK subsidiary of Pacific Dunlop and already the actual manufacturer of Mates. In return, Ansell had to pledge annual royalty payments and an advance-ment of one million pounds to the charity, which worked worldwide to educate about health issues.

SAFE AND SEXY

By 1988, Britons were using more than 140 million condoms a year, at a cost of over thirty-three million pounds. It was also the first choice in con-traception for married couples, turning around the 1960s trend of "pill only." By the early nineties, however, the STD numbers were once again on the rise, which moved the British Safety Council to call for a National Condom Week beginning in 1991; the first week featured the slogan "Slip into something safe and sexy," hoping to make condom use about intimacy as well as disease prevention. It is still an important part of the ongoing campaign against the spread of STDs, and has been sponsored by Durex since 1997.

HOT RUBBER

AIDS was a little slower to hit western Europe than the United States or the United Kingdom, but by the 1990s, Europe had in many ways surpassed the rest of the world in its efforts to combat the disease. Though each country has its own recent history in regards to just how it handled the new threat, overall there was considerably less politicization of the marketing and educating about the condom. Even most of the predominantly Catholic nations took little heed of the Church's insistence that the only safe sex was no sex. And as could probably be expected, the Scandinavian countries took the bull by the horns and made

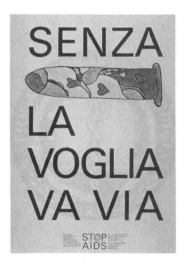

SENZA
LA
VOGLIA
VA VIA

STOP
AIDS

1980s Italian AIDS campaign poster

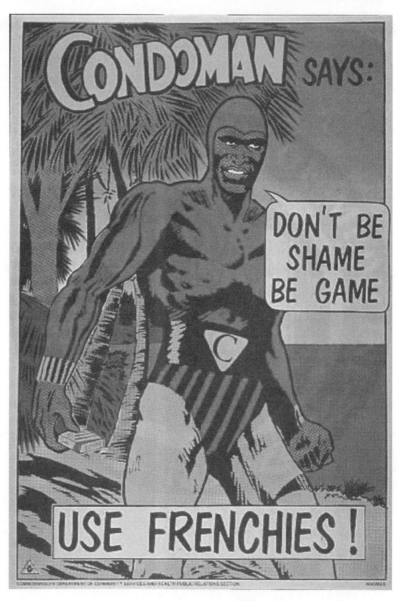

Australian AIDS campaign poster

kondoms, gummis, kondomis, and *kumis* readily available, no questions asked, a policy credited for their low incidence of AIDS.

That said, by the mid-eighties France was listed as third in number of reported cases of AIDS in Europe; Germany was sixth. By the early nineties, Spain had overtaken them, mainly because it had so many intravenous drug users, but no nation was immune. By mid-2005, there were 230,117 cases of HIV reported in twenty-one western European countries, a figure that the United Nations and other agencies question as so many cases may have gone and continue to go undiagnosed or

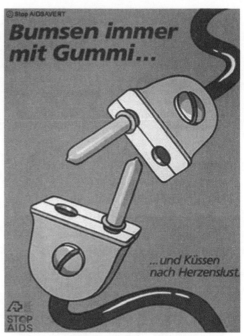

German AIDS campaign poster: *"Always screw with a rubber . . . and kiss to your heart's content."*

unreported. Spain, for instance, still has no national reporting system, Italy does not require that all regions report their cases, and France did not begin a national reporting system until the mid-2000s.

The Swiss, like the Scandinavians, were very proactive when it came to pushing the safe-sex message, and the least squeamish in their approach. In 1985 the Swiss AIDS Foundation actually established its own brand of condom, Hot Rubber, to sell solely to gay men. The point was to target just that group, with a campaign that sought to make condoms cheap and readily available and to remove the age-old stigma and embarrassment of buying and using them.

In the same year Hot Rubbers were introduced, sales went from two thousand the first month, to seventy-five thousand at the end of the year. Interestingly, by the nineties, Switzerland was considered the most suc-

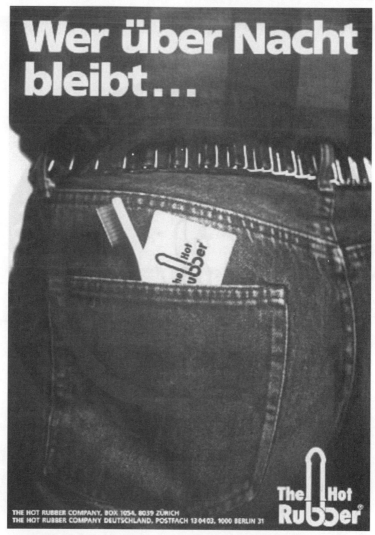

German AIDS campaign poster: "Anyone who stays overnight . . ."

IT'S NOT FRANCO'S SPAIN ANYMORE

By 1997 Spain had the highest incidence of AIDS anywhere in the European Union: 120,000 cases or one quarter of all infections. The Spanish Foundation Against AIDS responded by taking action at the grassroots level, targeting the nation's pride and joy, the Prado museum, as their first venue. Volunteers handed out post-cards with the slogan "Prevention is also an art," printed boldly below the image of Goya's The Nude Maja, along with two free condoms to each taker. Tourists expressed surprise at such a public campaign in a Catholic country, but thanks to the combined efforts of the Spanish government and the many agencies dedicated to prevention, the Spanish had purchased 120 million condoms, many more than ever before. As for the Church, when a nun hotly refused her free Prado con-doms then tried to convince two teenaged girls to return theirs, the girls politely declined.

cessful country in the world when it came to educating about condom use. That fact is due to a number of reasons, but perhaps the most signifi-cant is the marketing strategy used by the AIDS campaign, backed by the Swiss govern-ment. Unlike other countries, whose PSAs tried to second-guess just what citizens knew and understood about the dis-ease, the Swiss campaign sought to create messages that actually educated the adult population in a well-rounded, thorough manner. They avoided sensationalist lan-guage, cartoon caricatures, and scare tactics, and focused on

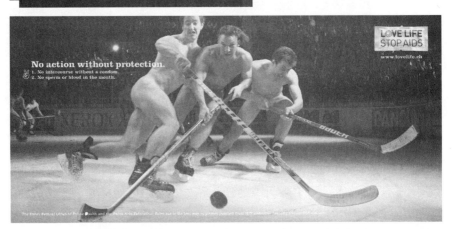

Swiss Love Life AIDS campaign (from the Love Life Stop AIDS campaign 2006 of the Swiss Federal Office of Public Health and the Swiss AIDS Federation).

GAY SLANG, 1950s–1980s
'50s: *Protective raincoat, Safety, Topcoat*
'60s–'80s: *Membranous envelopes, Come-
drum, Bag envelope, Love envelope,
Overcoat, Pecker glove, Apex envelopes,
Fibrous envelopes, French secret*

THE MODERN FEMALE CONDOM
Although the pessary in its many forms has been around for thousands of years, the first modern women's condom was introduced in Switzerland in 1992. It works on the same principle as the male, but is larger and, to some, not quite as "attractive" to use; although its sales pale in comparison with that of the male variety, it has gradually made its way around the world and is increasingly becoming part of international and local agencies' arsenal against AIDS. Some believe that it is the wave of the future, helping to empower women, especially in the developing world.

---

building on information and dispelling old chestnuts about condom use, along with encouraging listeners and viewers to understand that communication between partners was the key to comfort and safety.

From the onset of the first campaign to 1996, sales of condoms soared by 80 percent and the national symbol for the Swiss AIDS campaign, a rolled-up condom, had a 90 percent recognition factor.

And true to the history of sexually transmitted disease and the humble

---

PSAs AND "PROTECTION OF YOUR GOODS"
Of all the public service announcements working to educate the public about AIDS, one from Ghana may take the prize for the most metaphorical. Children were pictured playing in the rain, with a voiceover of:

> *When storms come, you need some protection for your goods. But the rain can be difficult and rain clothes can be most helpful (children shown playing in rain). They like to enjoy the fun and play in the rain. They don't feel threatened.*
>
> *Just as you protect your goods from the rain, protect your life against the disease AIDS.*
>
> *Like the rainstorm, the AIDS storm is here.*
> *Let's help fight it.*
> *Love with care. Stop AIDS. Don't be careless, get protection.*
> *National AIDS Control Programme, Ghana.*

---

little condom, even in this most efficient of nations, these successes would have their limits.

SPEAKING LIPS—A SWISS PSA

> *Man: I don't use condoms; they're not safe anyway.*
> *Woman: I don't need condoms. I make love only with healthy people.*
> *Man: Why would I use condoms? I'm not gay.*
> *Woman: I'm on the pill.*
> *Man: I don't need condoms because, well...*
> *Woman: French letters—they're embarrassing.*
> *Man: Rubbers? They ruin the whole mood.*
> *Man: We do use condoms because it's still the best protection against AIDS.*
> *Narrator: You know what's gonna happen, and make sure you have your rubber on. Stop AIDS!*

CHEEKY SCOTS AND THE CANNES FILM FESTIVAL

Germany's first-ever commercial television advertisement was aired in 1995, as a part of Durex's international advertising campaign on MTV, which eventually reached forty-nine million young adults in thirty-seven countries. MTV was the obvious choice for the campaign, since it was intended to reach a young, urban market; they chose the trendy, teen-oriented media outlet to make it clear "that condoms are fun.... We want to be seen as positive." The first in the series of ads, "Feeling Is Everything," featured a very sexy (some reviewers referred to it as "raunchy") scene involving a blind man and his lover. This was complemented with high-visibility billboards, and what marketing experts call "on-the-ground" activities—handing out freebies—and even providing condom machines with gratis provisions at the Cannes Film Festival, the European Music Awards, and the Vienna Life Ball, to mention a few.

For ten days that same year, a record-breaking thirty-meter (one-hundred-foot) -long condom flew over Italy's Adriatic coast to bring attention to a national anti-AIDS campaign, sponsored by the Italian gay and lesbian associations Arcigay and Arcilesbica. This was part of the launch of one of the biggest Italian anti-AIDS campaigns since the onset of the syndrome, and was condemned by the Vatican, which considered it an "official promotion of contraception" and "anti-educational and harmful to young people."

In 1997 a handful of cheeky Scottish health officials broke copyright by borrowing from a famous Levi Strauss–sponsored safe-sex ad. The original Levi's 501 commercial was shot in black and white, showing a teenager in a 1920s village buying a box of condoms from the local chemist, tucking one into his front pocket, only to be greeted at his girlfriend's door by the same chemist. The caption: "The Watch Pocket, created in 1873. Abused ever since." The Scots changed the caption to read: "Condoms. What to wear when you're not wearing jeans." Levi's loved it and gave its blessing for the doctored ad to be shown from "Munich to Madrid," eventually making it all the way to Asia.

That same year, while it made its way across Europe as part of the ongoing sales campaign, the Durex hot air balloon did not meet with such a successful response; while flying over France it had to make a forced landing in Belfort, within the walls of an enclosed order of nuns. Casanova, at least, would have approved.

And perhaps in the most global move to date, in 1997, Durex went modern with the first-ever commercial condom Web site.

WE ARE NOT AMUSED . . .

In 1999, Durex continued to roll out new styles just for the European market; its Comfort brand, meant for men between twenty-five and forty-five years of age who felt the older varieties were too "form fitting," was launched with an expensive media blitz. The commercials used the theme of "restricted space," like steamy sex in a steamier shower. They were well received in Italy and Spain, and moved on to Belgium and other European countries.

QUOTABLE QUOTES

"Using condoms is like listening to a symphony with cotton in your ears."

Author unknown

"Condoms aren't completely safe. A friend of mine was wearing one and got hit by a bus."

Bob Rubin

"There's a new medical crisis. Doctors are reporting that many men are having allergic reactions to latex condoms. They say they cause severe swelling. So where's the problem?"

Dustin Hoffman

"It is said that President Carter is considering changing the Democratic Party emblem from a jackass to a condom because it stands for inflation, protects a bunch of pricks, halts production, and gives a false sense of security while one is being screwed."

Anonymous, reported by Reinhold Aman, *Maledicta*, 1978

"My message to the businessmen of this country when they go abroad on business is that there is one thing above all they can take with them to stop them catching AIDS . . . and that is the wife."

Edwina Currie, *hot*, 1987

"Cheaper by the Dozen 2 is an argument for the cinematic equivalent of condoms."

David Germain, the Associated Press

A man walks into a drug store with his thirteen-year-old son. They happen to walk by the condom display, and the boy asks, "What are these, Dad?" To which the man matter-of-factly replies, "Those are called condoms, son. . . . Men use them to have safe sex."

"Oh I see," replied the boy pensively. "Yes, I've heard of that in health class at school." He looks over the display and picks up a package of three and asks, "Why are there three in this package?"

The dad replies, "Those are for high school boys. One for Friday, one for Saturday, and one for Sunday."

"Cool!" says the boy. He notices a six-pack and asks, "Then who are these for?"

"Those are for college boys." The dad answers, "TWO for Friday, TWO for Saturday, and TWO for Sunday."

"WOW!" exclaimed the boy, "then who uses THESE?" he asks, picking up a twelve-pack!

With a sigh, the dad replied, "Those are for married men. One for January, one for February, one for March . . ."

Perhaps the most controversial of the ads of the nineties was one produced by the British Safety Council. It featured a wedding photo of Prince Charles and Princess Diana on the balcony of Buckingham Palace kissing, with the caption: "Appearances can be deceptive. Use a Johnny Condom." The campaign began right after the princess had admitted to having an affair with her son's riding coach, and it was yanked immediately after its debut, presumably because of the queen's outrage at such an affront to the royal dignity.

The Europeans, on the other hand, were not shocked; the Norwegian Association for Sexual Information borrowed it and took out huge, two-page newspaper ads in some of Norway's most popular tabloids. The caption read: "It is very difficult to tell whether a person has had sex with casual partners. This happens in the best of families, so one cannot be too careful. More and more people regard a proposition for unprotected sex as an insult. A royal insult, indeed."

THE NORWEGIAN PREROGATIVE

The Norwegians are credited with creating a truly unique environment in regard to unmarried sexual encounters: it is considered an insult for a man not to use a condom when having sex with any partner to whom he is not married.

THE ROWDIEST OF ADS

By the late nineties, Lifestyle had run an ad campaign featuring fun and flirting with "Condoms shaped for two," Durex "Get one or get none" ads, and these were generally well received, but when Trojans tried to launch its "Blue balls" ads, the media said no. The ad used well-placed bright blue balls as the visual explanation for the young basketball player's collapse on the gym floor. The pretty cheerleader on the other side of the gym was the reason for his state. Although only a mature audience would understand the reference, the ads were considered to have gone too far.

Perhaps the most daring ad was the one run in Australia, which featured a nun holding out her hand, a rolled condom on her palm with the caption "Not on, Mate." It was pulled because of complaints, and picked up again in the mid-2000s, used in an anti-AIDS campaign in Taipei, Taiwan.

WHAT WOULD THE MRS. P'S THINK?
CONDOM CONGLOMERATES
AND THE GLOBAL ECONOMY

By the 1980s, when it came to condom manufacturing, a score card was required to figure out just who was making what for which market. The bad old days of living in fear of the law, peddlers in the parks, cutting out gut on the kitchen table, and glass penis molds were not even a dim memory in the life of the modern device. Gone was the brown paper package and the "little something for the weekend." And as usual, there were some unique personalities involved.

NOT SO GREEN

A major US university found that condoms make a considerable contribution to pollution in the United States and around the world. Because so many users enjoy having sex al fresco or in cars, they choose not to take the used protection with them and tend to leave the little items behind. Any serious runner will tell you how many can be seen while jogging along sidewalks, the sides of roads, and in parks. These often find their way into waterways and can be consumed by wildlife, who mistake the items for worms or other edibles.

In the 1980s, there were four dominant firms manufacturing and selling condoms in the United States. These sold about five hundred million units a year, 40 percent of those sold to the US government for free distribution via nongovernmental organizations working in the developing world (and sold at such a cut-rate price, they represented only about $15 million a year), but the rest were sold through the retail domestic market where they fetched a tidy sum.

Although small brands continued to show up both in the West and around the world, and some governments built subsidized factories in order to make cheap and plentiful rubbers, the industry continued to grow, diversify, buy, and sell—it continues to do so today.

TROJANS ARE TO CONDOMS
WHAT KLEENEX IS TO TISSUES

Trojan is surely the poster child for the modern history of the condom; when disaster hit, the industry geared up to the meet the need, and benefited handsomely from the effort. Merle Youngs's brainchild, and perhaps the most interesting and long-lasting example of the importance of brand names in the industry, continues to be very popular in the United States, Canada, and around the world.

Youngs had pioneered the concept of selling his top brand through a single source—the pharmacy—and until the AIDS scare pushed for expanded product availability and placement, that philosophy worked for Trojans throughout the twentieth century.

In 1985, a year after Youngs's Rubber won its second major case in court—the Supreme Court—the company decided to sell to Ansell, the huge Australian rubber manufacturer; the Justice Department's Anti-Trust Division, however, nixed the sale for fear the already powerful maker of the Mates brand, with about 20 percent of the English market, and the Lifestyles brand, which held about 5 percent of the US market, would end fair trade practice, given that Trojans represented about 56 percent of the commercial US market at that time. The Anti-Trust Division was especially concerned about the impact such a huge market share—and potential for one industry leader to dictate prices—would have on the US Agency for International Development. The agency purchased its rubbers at very attractive prices, but that could change in a "free market" where a dominant force could make it a little less free, specifically when it came to pricing.

Instead, Youngs Rubber, now Youngs Drug Products, which had remained in the founder's family for almost ninety years, chose to sell to Carter-Wallace, another of America's oldest established businesses. Famous in nineteenth-century industry

> ## NEED A MENTOR?
> *Once purchased by Carter-Wallace, Mentor's original design was changed to make it cheaper to produce. Unfortunately, it was considered by experts in the prevention of AIDS to be one of the very best because of a unique design element: it had an adhesive around the opening that formed a watertight barrier that prevented leakage and slippage.*

history as the maker of Carter's Little Liver Pills, the company also manufactured the Class Act brand condom, along with Nair Hair Remover, Pearl Drops toothpaste, and Arm & Hammer Baking Soda.

After purchasing Trojan, the company continued to use Youngs's original and very successful marketing strategy—a sales force that sold directly to pharmacies—and Trojan maintained its market share throughout the 1980s. Determined to expand further into that market, Carter-Wallace also bought the Mentor brand from Circle, adding up to about 30 percent of condom sales in the United States and the United Kingdom, but raising no eyebrows with the anti-trust watchdogs.

By 2000 Trojan held an almost 69 percent share of the market, which made it a cash cow for Carter-Wallace and, with an ever-expanding market, an appealing deal for another, even bigger company. The British firm Church and Dwight purchased it (along with the other personal hygiene lines) in a package deal for $739 million. By 2001 its new owners knew they had made a good deal because the "condom category" had a "high growth potential." Again.

Although it never made much headway in the United Kingdom, Trojan remains America's favorite.

AND THEN THERE WAS JULIUS'S COMPANY

It would probably not have come as a big surprise to America's first condom king to find that, fifty years after his death, by the 1980s Schmid's enduring Ramses and Sheik were still very popular brands, holding about 34 percent of the American market share. Like their popular rival, that fact also made Schmid very attractive to those conglomerates itching to get their hands on already established brand names. What might have surprised both Merle and Julius is the way their prized possessions moved back and forth across the pond.

That other old brand, London Rubber Company, established by L. A. Jackson in 1915, had begun to manufacture its own brand, Durex, in 1932; prior to that, it had purchased its rubbers from German firms. By 1950 it was trading on the London Stock Exchange, the same year it had begun to sell its London and Hatu brands in Europe. In 1961, taking advantage of the

CREATIVE NAMES, POST-1981
The names given to rubber brands, the most creative emerging after the mideighties, boggle the mind, and certainly make the historical lexicon of the condom seem quite tame. To name only a few: Aegis Big Boy, Banana Hit, Rulex Rony Wrinkle, Snug Fit, Skin, Sweet Rider, Cool, Gold Circle, Double-Butterfly, Kimono, Tahiti, Arouse, Embrace Her, They-Fit, Crown, Beyond Seven, Paradise, Sagami, Female, Trustex, Madonna, KISS, Vivid, Prime, Contempo, Crowd Stopper, Joy, Frenzy, Hot Rod, HUGE . . . and in honor of a visit made to China by American President Bill Clinton, the Monica Lewinsky (Laiwensifi) and Clinton (Kelitun).

THE NEW OLD VENDOR
Although there was nothing new about the vending machines themselves, new research had proved that first-time condom buyers got their "taste" for the devices they would otherwise be too embarrassed to buy.

emerging Indian market, it ventured into that country, too. In 1962 it purchased Julius Schmid, Inc., merging in the mideighties to become the London International Company. All was not rosy on the condom front by that period, however, as the company's American director began to diversify into murky markets, which meant the lifelong focal point of both London Rubber and Schmid—condoms—was set aside as this director purchased new, unrelated product lines, landing London International in the red.

When new management stepped in to try to save the company, they decided to bring its focus back to condoms, and only condoms. It did not stop there. Although London International's Durex enjoyed the lion's share of the British market well into the 1990s, the company also launched the first really new condom in many years; the Avanti was made of polyurethane, which was half the thickness and had twice the strength of the latex variety, and was intended for those who were allergic to or sensitive to latex. They went under the Schmid label in the United States, and helped put the company back on the map, as did the acquisition of the Protex brand, a subsidiary of Allercare, which gave Schmid a toehold in the vending machine market, a first for the company.

With all the buying came some selling, and the decision was made to tighten up production and brand-name use. In an early example of offshoring, some English manufacturing facilities were shut in order to save money and replaced with factories in Malaysia, Thailand, and India, which made the business lean and mean—and very profitable. Durex remained on top of the English market, along with a handsome share of markets around the world. It enjoyed healthy sales to the US Agency for International Development, purchased the Malaysian brand Mister (marketed in Europe), the Spanish brand Androtex, the US Aladan Corporation, as well as buying into joint ventures in China, and moving into the central and eastern European, Russian, and Latin American markets. It also launched the biggest international condom advertising campaign ever. London International was so successful that none other than the global magnet George Soros bought a lot of its valuable stock.

ANTI-TRUST, ENGLISH-STYLE

There had been concern on the part of the English government's Monopolies and Mergers Commission about then London International Group's grip on the condom market in the United Kingdom even before the boon in sales by the mideighties, but had tacitly supported it in order to keep National Health Services' sheaths cheap. By the late nineties, it was a new day and new brands were trying to make inroads into that market, leading the same body to realize that it needed to limit the company's practice of forcing retailers and wholesalers into exclusive supply agreements. Competition might mean an even cheaper public supply. It had taken almost twenty years, the AIDS scare, and Mates' high visibility to finally end Durex's stranglehold, but even then, it remained the overwhelming favorite . . . partly due to its longevity, partly because of its history.

Sadly, though, by the late nineties Sheik, Ramses, and the other Schmid brands held only 20 percent of the overall American market, leading the company to decide to eliminate those brands, morphing them into one: Durex. This consolidation success led the company's head to wonder why all LCI products had not borne the label Durex from the start. After all, "We want to be like Coke or Gillette." Schmid's lifelong labors, on the other hand, became a footnote in the history of the device.

The conglomerate saga was not over yet, however, when an unlikely business came looking to expand into the condom market.

> **GOOD VIBES**
> By the 2000s, the device had gone high tech, to include designs that were meant to double up as vibrators.

As a medical student at the beginning of the twentieth century, in order to pay his tuition William Scholl had worked in a shoe store, an experience that had convinced him badly fitting shoes caused a great deal of pain and discomfort for many. This led him to focus all his efforts on opening a shop dedicated to foot care. Over the years, his creativity in developing popular remedies and his ability to merchandise meant that Dr. Scholl's turned into a profitable corporation, but it would perhaps have come as a shock to the company's founder, a simple man born on a dairy farm in Indiana, had he lived to see his beloved company enter into the sexual aides business.

By the late nineties, Dr. Scholl's Foot Care had merged its European line with the English firm Seton Healthcare Group, forming Seton Scholl Healthcare. They in turn purchased London International Limited; together they became Seton Scholl Limited (SSL), one of the world's largest commercial condom enterprises.

THE DUNLOP PNEUMATIC TYRE COMPANY

Like the other major condom manufacturers, Ansell, a division of Pacific Dunlop Corporation, had very humble origins. Dunlop was opened by and named after the inventor of the pneumatic tire, John Boyd Dunlop, a Scottish veterinary surgeon who lived and worked in Belfast, Ireland, and whose work in the late 1880s was recognized as an important innovation for the bike, and later, the car industry. When his invention was exported to Australia in 1889, it was very well received, encouraging the Dunlop company to open an outlet in Melbourne. In spite of its successes, however, the parent company had financial difficulties early on and sold off some of its branches, including its Melbourne interest. This was purchased by a Canadian syndicate, which renamed the business the Dunlop Pneumatic Tyre Company of Australasia, Ltd. The name Dunlop had stuck.

In the 1890s the original company had done what many rubber companies had done, and diversified by manufacturing condoms for the Australian market. The new company, however, decided against continuing this end of the business, and in 1905 gave the condom-making equipment to an employee of the company—Eric Ansell—who called his new endeavor the Ansell Rubber Company. Many years later, in 1969, that company ended up being sold back to the Dunlop Company. Today, this mega-company's brands include Goodyear, Wonderbra, Tropicana, Hanes, and Jockey, to name only a few.

Still in the condom business, Ansell has done well with Richard Branson's brainchild, the Mates brand, and under the Ansell-America's label, the company also produces the popular Lifestyle brand, which by the mideighties held only 5 percent of the US and Canadian market, but gained strides after extensive marketing campaigns by the late nineties. Because of those successes, the company added "subbrands" to its lines, like Canadian labels Kama Sutra, Contempo, and Discs; in Europe, Mates were labeled Maxix in France, Akuel in Italy, and Primex in Spain; in Australia and New Zealand, they were Chekmate and Affinity. By the mid-2000s, Ansell, with all of its international concerns, was a many-billion-dollar concern.

Other manufacturers abounded, like Japan's number one company Okamoto, which maintained a distant fourth place in the American market; Britain's Pasante Healthcare with a small retail presence, but specializing in providing to the National Health Services; Condom Solutions Limited, which distributed condoms to university student union shops and vending machines; and the German Condomi, with its bright pink in-store kiosks—to name only a few. Then, between government and nonprofit organizations' efforts, countries like Thailand, Malaysia, India, and many others had their own plants, as well as generic exports from the West's biggest producers, a number of whom maintained huge production facilities in those and other countries, making massive numbers of inexpensive, and not necessarily very high-quality, condoms per year. In fact, when the profits from sales of "no names" to those agencies were factored in to the retail sales of name brands, the net worth of the humble little condom by the end of the 1990s boggles the mind.

A STRANGE SUCCESS STORY

Because of the huge surge in demand for rubber, by the late 1980s Liberia's rubber plantations were doing a booming business as they tried to meet the international demand for 60,000 tons of latex a year. Consistent with the history of disease and prevention, the disease that would eventually mean doom and gloom to the African continent enriched one of America's oldest and most successful industries on that same continent. Firestone Corporation planted the huge Liberian rubber plantations, which they still own, in 1926, complete with a company town named after the owner and his wife—Harvey and Idabelle—"Harbel." Since the 1980s, more than 2 percent of the world's rubber, used to make high-quality latex condoms, has come from Firestone's plantation. Although the company is careful to couch its successes as gains for Liberia and its people, it has for years faced accusations of slavery on its plantations. As for AIDS, by 2003, almost 6 percent (100,000) of the population was living with HIV/AIDS, and there were 36,000 children who had been orphaned because of the disease.

THAT MOST CATHOLIC OF NATIONS . . .
THE CASE OF IRELAND

> *The Irish Government, while holding the EC presidency as a*
> *Western democracy, appear to treat their citizens with the same*
> *disregard as Ceausescu did in Romania.*
>
> Richard Branson, 1991

When it came to condoms, no other country could compete with Ireland's resistance to their use. In spite of the fact that it was legal to marry at the age of sixteen, and even after the highly visible international campaigns about the prevention of AIDS, by the late eighties, over-eighteen-year-old married men and women could only obtain prevention from a government-licensed clinic or chemist.

True to his activist spirit, Richard Branson assisted the Irish Family Planning Association to challenge that fact; in his Dublin Virgin Mega-store, under the sign "Irish Family Planning Association," that daring group set up a kiosk to sell Mates condoms, which of course was illegal. They managed to work under the radar screen of the local authorities until very conservative groups pushed the local Garda to close down the kiosk. When Detective Sergeant John McKeown walked into the Virgin store, he bought a packet of three, charged the group with breaching the 1985 Family Planning Act, and fined them four hundred Irish pounds. This seemingly simple act actually got the attention of the foreign press, and newspapers around the world decryed the oppressive laws of the Irish Republic. It also brought U2's Bono into the condom controversy—he and his band paid the fine and, in defiance of the law, the kiosk stayed open.

The rest of the story is farcical at best, but the up-and-coming Irish capital, with its vibrant universities, night life, and increasingly European mentality, saw many Irishmen defying the law. A variety of courageous businesses and private interests continued on with what the family planning group had begun; they placed vending machines in student unions, pubs, and social clubs, and the government was forced to change the laws, crawling toward condom acceptance. Not, however, before tens of thousands of people contracted HIV/AIDS, and the continuing struggle over birth control left a lot of Irishmen—and women—miserable.

THE BATTLE OVER BIRTH CONTROL

It was after Ireland's fight for freedom that it became the West's most sexually oppressed nation. The 1937 Constitution was meant to meld Catholic ideology with government principle; the 1968 papal encyclical "Humanae Vitae" had banned artificial contraception, a policy that acted as a guiding light, and excuse, for the Irish government to maintain its ban against birth control. Many of the Irish, however, had a different idea. By 1974 at least forty thousand Irish women were on the Pill and at least ten million condoms were being sold per year—all "black market" or smuggled in. In tacit recognition of this clash between public and private practice, the Health Bill of 1978 included a section on family planning and allowed for limited availability, but it was too little too late, especially when the AIDS virus hit the little nation; it was not until 1993 that all restrictions on condom sales were lifted, ten years after the first reported cases of AIDS in Ireland.

WHO OBJECTED? RECYCLING THE DEBATE

Surgeon General Koop was not without his critics, especially when he came straight out with the message that no amount of adult education would eradicate the new disease without also bringing the safe-sex message to public schools: "We need sex education in schools and ... it must include information on heterosexual and homosexual relationships."

Public polls had for years shown that the American public, or at least over 80 percent of it, agreed with the good doctor. But there were still those who objected, some on religious grounds, others with their own agendas. Right after Koop's public education statement, Catholic leaders announced that the Church's ban on condoms "has not been modified in light of the AIDS epidemic and it will not be ... America is bound and determined to make sex as casual and unsupportive as shaking hands," and "We believe that condoms, by promoting immoral sexual behavior, are actually accelerating the spread of AIDS. ... The efficacy of condoms is questionable. Their use gives people a false sense of security." Then there was that great moral scion Phyllis Schlafly—who declared that teaching children about condoms was immoral because, "It's the cause of promiscuity and destroys the natural modesty of girls"—along with a less public mix of naysayers, made up of antiabortionists, homophobes, and even those who wanted a piece of the action when it came to public school health clinics (and their potential profits), who made up the anticondom-in-public-schools lobby.

THE CASE OF THE MISSING KETCHUP

In 2005 a leading member of the Mormon Church in Utah received a panicked call from a parishioner of his temple, demanding he join a large group of parents from the same temple in their protest against the local McDonald's. The source of the woman's rage? The restaurant was offering free condoms with any purchase!

When the leader arrived to check it out for himself, he realized what the problem was. The sign hanging in the window read: "Free condiments with any purchase."

If I could be the "condom queen" and get every young person who
engaged in sex to use a condom in the United States, I would wear
a crown on my head with a condom on it! I would!

Surgeon General Joycelyn Elders

It was in this strange atmosphere of battling pros and cons that America's most plain-speaking surgeon general since Thomas Parran took her place in the new president's cabinet; the condom was front and center when President Bill Clinton chose Joycelyn Elders as his surgeon general, becoming not only the first woman but the first African American to hold the office. Her initial public appearance with Clinton had actually been while he was governor of Arkansas, also Elder's home state, and she was his appointed director of health. When asked by a reporter if Elders supported making contraceptives available to teens in Arkansas schools and she responded with "We're not going to put condoms on their lunch trays, but yes," it left both Clinton and the reporter pink faced. Perhaps Bill should have seen the writing on the walls.

Elders entered office with a broad and, to some, a shocking, agenda: she was determined to keep abortion legal, make sex education mandatory for all school-aged children, legalize the morning-after pill, and she wanted every middle and high school student to have free and easy access to condoms in school. Her high-profile, no-holds-barred public persona offended conservative politicians and their constituents who, like so many of their forebears, did not want this kind of sexual openness and made it their business to assure that this public servant's time in office would have a very short shelf life.

Our children have seen 15,000 hours of TV to only 11,000 hours
of reading, writing, and arithmetic. We've not used the most
powerful medium—that's our television—to educate our people
[against AIDS]. That says our country has really not made a
commitment.

Surgeon General Joycelyn Elders
United Nations, World AIDS Day, December 1, 1994

In spite of Koop's courage and outreach to the American public, by the mid-1990s, Elders knew the numbers indicated that all was not working when it came to preventing sexually transmitted diseases. Although the condom marketers were shifting their focus in order to respond to the surging numbers of many STDs, the new surgeon general felt that the American government was not even coming close to using its immense potential to influence and educate the public about safer sex. Elders believed that education and availability were the answers to the STD and unwanted-pregnancy problems of the United States and was the first to point out what she said was "obvious": in nations where sex education began in the classroom, there were far fewer abortions, and the United States could have solved once and for all both concerns by facing the issues with honesty and practicality.

That strident approach to these terminally prickly issues put her in the eye of a public storm—and in spite of his support for increasing funding for research and to help the victims of AIDS, President Clinton was not willing to spend precious political capital on a cabinet member the press had quickly dubbed the "condom queen."

After only fifteen months in office, Elders was dismissed as surgeon general when she stated publicly that children should be educated to masturbate in order to avoid STDs. That was the straw that broke the camel's back.

❈❈❈

> *AIDS will definitely change the nature of sex education as we*
> *know it. . . . It will lead to more open, explicit discussions about*
> *condoms and other strategies for safe sex. Though we are at a*
> *point where sex education is no longer a matter of morals—it's a*
> *matter of life and death.*
> Harvey Fineberg, dean of the Harvard School of Public Health

Not surprising given Elders's experiences, in spite of the many polls indicating that an overwhelming number of American parents felt that some sort of sex education should be offered to middle and high school students, the Centers for Disease Control and Prevention reported that even by the

2000s only 70 percent of middle schools and 85 percent of high schools provided any information about STDs in or out of the classroom. There was no national curriculum available to the schools, and what little was offered was driven solely by local school boards; even in California, considered one of the most liberal of the states, the law required only one class in both middle and high school that was to cover STDs—less than two hours of education in the life of a public school child. The chances of those classes containing any information at all on condom use was very unlikely, and most offered only watered-down "lessons" squeezed into science or health classes. Rarely, too, were they taught by teachers with any training in the area of sex ed; in fact, teachers who were polled regarding their approach to teaching safe sex revealed that only a tiny percentage of them were comfortable in talking about sex to their students.

There were only a handful of high schools, all in major cities, which offered clinics where students could receive counseling and condoms; when George W. Bush came into office, these already underfunded sites came under greater and greater pressure to teach abstinence only. No condoms, no straight talk about disease.

It seemed by the early 2000s, the condom had come full circle . . . again.

In the case of the United Kingdom and Europe, although many English schools have offered sex education since the 1990s, some as early as primary school, the argument continued through that decade and into the 2000s as to whether to make learning about safer sex compulsory: the lack of political will to push that message, along with limited free or cheap condom access—and no standardized curriculum—have been blamed for the high teen-pregnancy rate and, by the late nineties, an ever-increasing STD rate, especially pronounced in the fifteen- to twenty-four-year age range.

Europeans, some as early as the

> ## SEX ON THE BEACH
> *By the late nineties, it was discovered that one out of every six British tourists between the ages of eighteen and thirty-two had sex with someone he or she had just met while on vacation, and only half of those used condoms.*

THE SPRAY-ON KIND

Scientists at the Institute for Condom Consultancy—really!—in Germany are developing a spray-on condom. A spokesmen said that it will be perfect for men of all sizes: "We're trying to develop the perfect condom for men that's suited to every size of penis. . . . We're very serious." The man using it must insert his member into a spray can, press a button, and on goes a painted condom. They will also come in many colors.

Not to be outdone, the German firm Lebenslust (Lust for Life) designed a computer program which makes a 3D image of a man's privates, and the company then designs the perfect gummi for him. Cost? The service runs about $1,200 for the image, pattern, and an unspecified number of the items. Customers may also have them engraved with their names.

1980s, on the other hand, have realized the benefits of early and hard-hitting sex ed, and they have some of the lowest STD and teen-pregnancy rates in the world. Interestingly, Sweden led the way in this effort, and began its successful sex education push long before the AIDS scare, in an attempt to protect its youth from the other STDs and teen pregnancy. The Swedish success story is explained by the United Nations International Children's Emergency Fund:

> Recommendations of abstinence were dropped and sex only within marriage were dropped, contraceptive education was made explicit, and a nationwide network of youth clinics was established specifically to provide confidential contraceptive advice and free contraceptives.

As the nineties, and disease, progressed, even Sweden was not immune, and the government and private and public agencies refurbished their long-standing philosophy: by the end of the decade, they saw another 40 percent drop in the national STD rate, which had never been high.

Other European countries—the Netherlands, for instance—believe that their successes have been due to very open discussion of sexuality, the lack of shame involved in asking questions about the subject or in buying condoms, and the media's willingness to "tell it like it is" in commercial and publicly sponsored ads. All of these have enhanced the countrywide public school efforts.

NOW YOU CAN GET **12 FREE** CONDOMS (Rubbers) WITH YOUR MEDICAL ASSISTANCE CARD ASK YOUR PHARMACIST

Supported by:
Maryland Society of Hospital Pharmacists
Maryland Pharmaceutical Association
An educational grant provided by Ansell,
maker of Lifestyle Condoms.

HITTING THE HIGH NOTE

A musical condom designed to play louder and faster as lovers reach a climax is being marketed in the Ukraine. These come with a special sensor that registers when the item is put on, then it transmits a signal to a tiny speaker at the base, which will play a melody.

A company representative told reporters that: "As the sex becomes more passionate, it registers the increased speed of the movements and plays the melody faster and louder."

THE ANTIRAPE CONDOM

A South African inventor, Sonette Ehlers, developed an antirape female condom, which debuted in Cape Town, South Africa, in the late 1980s. The purpose was to help cut down on sexual assaults, which were the highest in the world at that time. It was meant to hook onto an attacker's penis, making it too painful to proceed with the attack. Sadly, probably because of a lack of monies for marketing and distribution, or perhaps because of design flaws, it did not catch on.

THE GRAMEEN OF SHEATHS . . . THE REST OF THE WORLD

AIDS was slow to reach the developing nations, but when it did, the effects were devastating. There were of course countries like Bangladesh and Afghanistan, whose leaders for years into the epidemic absolutely refused to admit that there were any cases of AIDS at all in those troubled nations. But, as in the case of Bangladesh, the early US-led birth control movement, begun in the 1960s as the West's answer to the East's population explosion, had at least begun the process of creating an infrastructure for the distribution of condoms and education about condom use.

I don't find this odd at all, but a lot of people do. I mean, what else would I do with the money? This is my life's work. I can't think of any more enjoyable way to make use of these profits.
Philip Harvey, founder of DKT International
and owner of Adam and Eve

Philip Harvey, the cofounder of PSI, the mail-order company that in 1970 challenged the law in order to provide easy-access condoms to college students around the United States, was back in a big way by the late 1980s, when he founded his nonprofit, DKT International (named after an Indian birth control pioneer). Harvey had served with an aid agency in India during the 1960s, where he saw for himself just how vital a role the condom could play in limiting that country's burgeoning population; later he applied the same philosophy to the prevention of disease. But it is perhaps his talent for blending business and humanism that makes him a true pioneer.

Harvey is the founder of Adam and Eve, America's most successful sex-aid business, which began life as a condom catalog but soon branched out into all kinds of toys. From his sexy $70 million yearly sales, he contributed (and still does) to his nonprofit to help people in the developing world practice safe sex and birth control. His intent was to make inexpensive condoms available to people in ten developing nations. This philosophy makes him a pioneer in the new breed of "philanthropreneurs"—those successful young entrepreneurs-turned-philanthropists, which includes Richard Branson, Steve Jobs, and Pierre Omidijar, founders of Virgin, Apple Computer, and eBay (respectively), who use their profits and knowledge of business to help others to help themselves; Harvey used his very successful—and controversial—commercial business to fund his nonprofit efforts *and* he proved that his philosophy about the human spirit was correct. DKT provides millions of condoms, made in Asian factories or provided by USAID, a year, but with a slightly different

CREATIVE FUNDING

Harvey and his partner, Dr. Tim Black, actually came up with idea of how to fund their nonprofit idea during their early days as condom pioneers. The partners asked themselves "what if," by selling all those condoms to America's youth, they could generate enough cash to fund social-marketing projects overseas? They would be able to bypass traditional donors and operate with "liberating autonomy." The two christened the profit-making arm of their venture Population Planning Associates and set up a separate nonprofit, Population Services International (PSI), which by 1975 was running condom-marketing programs in Kenya and Bangladesh.

DURABLE DURIAN

DKT International works hard to meet the needs and tastes of its international recipients. They have even experimented with flavored condoms, to include using the durian fruit—popular in Vietnam—to make an interesting variety. The problem is that the durian fruit is very sweet and juicy . . . and has a foul-smelling rind, making it hard to make a sweet-tasting condom without it smelling terrible.

twist from the other nonprofits. They sell theirs. According to Harvey, "After thirty-five years in this business, I've never seen a giveaway program that worked very well for very long." Harvey knows that by charging even a few cents, those buying his condoms—mostly men—will feel they have a vested interest in actually using their purchases.

In Ethiopia, his organization has created a model that could save many lives in other countries; it has joined forces with the military, selling millions of condoms at no more than a penny apiece. Soldiers are required to carry one whenever they head off base; the program has helped keep that army's HIV infection rate to around 5 percent, believed to be the lowest on the continent. Many other African armies have rates as high as 30 to 40 percent.

And, like so many condom pioneers before him, Harvey has had to fight to keep DKT in the forefront of disease prevention, but the struggle has not been with third-world bureaucrats, but rather with American authorities. He risked losing

> ## MARIE STOPES INTERNATIONAL
> Dr. Tim Black, cofounder of PSI, picked up where Marie Stopes had left off. As an offshoot of Stopes's work in bringing birth control clinics to the United Kingdom, Black expanded on that idea and created the nonprofit Marie Stopes International, a large reproductive health organization, with branches all over the world. Black's early work in trying to supply young Americans with condoms is now one of the world's largest organizations of its type.

DKT's federal funding from USAID when he would not sign a pledge opposing prostitution and sex trafficking because as an equal opportunity condom proponent he did not want to be restricted from providing them to prostitutes; by signing the pledge, he would not be able to work with that vulnerable population. He also defied the federal government in the early nineties, when he kept his representatives in Haiti during a US embargo that squashed the distribution of condoms. His workers stayed on to ensure that condoms remained cheap and abundant.

Harvey's bottom line? Nothing new . . . "They are so simple and yet so effective. They're cheap, they work anywhere in the world, and they fit everybody."

EPILOGUE

plenty of condoms, no water

THE NEW MILLENNIUM

etween 1995 and 2004, government and private agencies from Western nations had donated more than sixteen billion condoms and over $652 million for purchase, production, and education about their use to developing nations. By the turn of the twenty-first century, the number and variety of condoms being produced and sold on the world retail market was staggering, the details of which would require many long chapters to describe, but just a sampling gives some idea as to the scope of the business that was once dominated by the "poor and disenfranchised," conducted "behind closed doors."

Consider that in the first six months of 2006, just in the United Kingdom, Durex sold ninety million pounds' worth of retail condoms; US sales went past the $444 million mark, and even in the little Philippines, a longtime no-condom zone because of the influence wielded by the Catholic Church, sales skyrocketed. In Europe, the Spanish purchased the greatest number—their favorite made in Japan—but in every European country, huge amounts of money were being exchanged in the sale and purchase of the little device.

But in the time of AIDS, it is perhaps the "other" numbers that tell the rest of story.

By the end of the 2000s, as contagion spread across the globe, millions upon millions were affected: in 1990, eight million people had the disease; in 2006, UNAIDS reported just under forty million victims. Add in all of the other STDs, most of which were on the rise again, and the plagues of the past pale in comparison. What went wrong?

There were those aid workers posted in the developing world who had the sense that there were "condoms condoms everywhere," leading one of them to complain that so much foreign aid had been diverted to the effort to prevent AIDS that desperately needed funds were not available for life-sustaining essentials like clean water: "We have plenty of condoms, but no clean water." Though there are not sufficient monies to meet all the needs of an increasingly stressed world, the notion that there are "too many condoms" is simply untrue. More numbers . . .

In the developing world, in spite of the huge number of condoms being distributed through local, national, and international efforts, with the ever-increasing populations of most countries, meaning a younger and younger population base, there simply have never been enough to go around. According to Population Action International, in 2002 alone, almost 2.5 billion condoms were distributed and a little over $76 million was provided for education and distribution. This was up from 950 million distributed in 2000.

That may have been a lot of aid and effort devoted to one little device, but the question is, what was actually needed?

In 2002, in order to have met the demands of the developing world, a total of 9.9 billion condoms, and $1.5 billion for education and distribution, would have been required. By 2015, it is predicted that the developing nations will need at least 18.6 billion condoms and over $2 billion in funding for education and distribution. And perhaps the aid worker frustrated with too many condoms and no clean water had a point in that there has been incredible focus on production and, to a lesser extent, distribution. Stopping AIDS, however, is so much more than a numbers game. Beyond the question of how many condoms can the world produce, or how much money the developed nations will or can provide, prevention is a much bigger issue. It is really about politics, culture, corruption, and the age-old arguments surrounding the "rights and wrongs" of human sexuality. These are, or should be, front and center in any discussion of the modern condom.

NO AIDS WHEN THE SUN GOES DOWN . . .

In spite of the large sums spent on distributing prevention to the poor, corruption at national and local levels means that the monies and devices provided by many of the leading aid agencies may or may not make it to their intended destinations, a fact that influenced the Bill and Melinda Gates Foundation to insist upon very tight reporting from any of the aid they provide to groups working on this issue. Then there are the tariffs and taxes charged on condoms either pilfered before arriving at their intended destination or given to "local authorities for local distribution," and intended to be free. Restrictive social norms and cultural strictures that make it difficult for young people to negotiate condom use, especially young women, who so often remain at the mercy of boys and men, also limit their use. Add to that the terrible plight of women in many African nations, where civil war and ethnic hatred put them in harm's way, where rape is a daily threat—no amount of latex is going to solve these overwhelming problems.

Where there are functional distribution systems, there are still the issues of poor or inadequate public education, confounded by low literacy rates and insufficient training. Trained educators can communicate the message in a culturally sensitive manner, which makes teaching about safer sex a tremendous challenge. Then there is the problem of "condom misinformation," some of which seems to follow the pattern of neighborhood legend—a fairly common one, reported by child sex workers in Liberia as their customers' excuse for refusing to wear protection, is that AIDS "goes away" after six PM, making condoms unnecessary "after the sun goes down"—and then there are the unconscionable public statements by those who should know better: the archbishop of Nairobi, Raphael Ndingi Nzeki, has preached against condom use, claiming "AIDS . . . has grown so fast because of the availability of condoms," while other clergymen in Africa borrowed yet another neighborhood legend to warn their parishioners not to use *soksi*, telling them that they were intentionally laced with the HIV virus at the factory.

When this is all placed into the context of the horrendous social, political, and economic upheavals being experienced around the world, it is little wonder why unprotected sex continues to infect millions. But just what is the West's excuse?

A WAR OF WORDS . . . MORAL PROPHYLAXIS IS BACK

In the late 1990s when former US presidential hopeful Bob Dole went on prime-time TV as the national spokesman for "erectile dysfunction medication," some optimistic advocates of an open and honest public dialogue about safer sex, including unrestricted advertising about and distribution of condoms, believed the time had finally come. Not quite.

Although there were no laws preventing advertising on prime time, many of the social barriers remained in place into the twenty-first century; the very first American condom commercials shown prior to eleven PM were for Trojans—in 2005. The ads were very sobering, using statistics to sell the public on the dangers of sex without protection, the kind of shock method the industry had abandoned years prior. The company's vice president of marketing described the approach: "Our statistics show that 15 million Americans each year contract STDS. We believe that the way we've communicated that is respectful and tasteful." But the increase in contagion in many Western nations cannot be blamed on the shortage of condom ads. The reasons are a complicated mix of a lack of coordinated effort, where commercial and public interests work together instead of the piecemeal efforts of the past; inadequate or inappropriate public school education about sexual health; the retail cost of condoms; and the continued stigma when it comes to buying them. Yet perhaps the problem goes even deeper.

Like eras past, by the turn of the twenty-first century, many people had become complacent, the issue having fallen off their radar screens, while others had "message fatigue." Then there were those who had entered the sexual scene after the first really high-visibility news stories and public service announcements had done their jobs in making the sexually active

THE VIAGRA C.
In 2005 a British company created a condom with an "erectogenic compound," responding the to concern that some men could not maintain their passion when interrupted to put on protection. The new device was supposed to help prevent slippage, thereby increasing enjoyment and providing protection . . . all in one. If the Viagra condom passes all the required tests, Durex plans to distribute it worldwide.

SHARP
In a response to a rise in AIDS and other STD cases, the US Navy's Sexual Health and Responsibility Program was that bureaucracy's attempt at promoting safe sex:

> *Often an emotionally-charged issue, targeted condom distribution efforts require thoughtful planning and leadership courage. Access strategies should be sensitive to community concerns and perceptions. Specific examples are discussed herein.*
> *Leadership support is essential.*

FDR might have been disappointed.

THE EUROPEAN MODEL
Europeans are far less squeamish, and EU nations responded to increases in STDs in the 2000s with vigor. In France, the government backed a plan to make condoms very inexpensive; in 2005, a pack of five could be purchased for one euro. Over half of French high schools sold them, and the government encouraged sales at hospitals, newspaper kiosks, nightclubs, and cinemas, as well as at more standard retail outlets. Whether the health minister knew that he was bringing back an old model or not, his plan did not include one element of the past efforts: a public debate over the morality of such a campaign.

afraid. Seniors, who had been monogamous for years before divorce or widowhood put them "out there" again, never thought of themselves as potential victims and were becoming vulnerable to contagions, as were younger and younger teens, who had had little or no exposure to the message from the mediums from which they received their information.

In the United States and the United Kingdom, minorities were disproportionately represented, leading AIDS activists to the conclusion that those groups had been left out of the net when it came to any real education on the subject of sex. Yet perhaps, not just for those two countries that are experiencing such dramatic increases in STDs, but for everyone, the challenge of actually getting people, generation after generation, to act responsibly, while at the same time, admitting that the human animal is a very sexual one, seems to get lost in the rhetoric, and too much energy goes to fighting the same old fight instead of admitting what that World War II army doctor had said to his men, which was really the bottom line: "Angels belong in heaven."

A SAMPLER OF THE WAR OF WORDS

Although sexual abstinence is a desirable objective, programs must include instruction in safer sex behavior, including condom use. The effectiveness of these programs is supported by strong scientific evidence.

The National Institutes of Health, 1997

The folks that are saying condom distribution is the best way to reduce teenage pregnancies obviously haven't looked at the statistics.

Presidential candidate George W. Bush, November 1999

Current research findings do not support the position that the abstinence-only approach to sexuality education is effective in delaying the onset of intercourse.

The American Medical Association, 1999

It's very important to understand the power and promise of abstinence education.

Presidential candidate George W. Bush, September 2000

All adolescents should be counseled about the correct and consistent use of latex condoms to reduce risk of infection.

American Academy of Pediatrics, January 2001

I simply wished to remind the public, seconding the opinion of a good number of experts, that when the condom is employed as a contraceptive, it is not totally dependable, and that the cases of pregnancy are not rare. In the case of the AIDS virus, which is around 450 times smaller than the sperm cell, the condom's latex material obviously gives much less security. These margins of uncertainty . . . should represent an obligation on the part of the health ministries and all these campaigns to act in the same way as they do with regard to cigarettes, which they state to be a danger.

Vatican Cardinal Alfonso Lopez Trujillo, 2003

These incorrect statements about condoms and HIV are dangerous when we are facing a global pandemic which has already killed more than 20 million people, and currently affects at least 42 million.

World Health Organization's response to Trujillo, 2003

A condom, when it is used for the protection of life, is not only a matter in the sexual domain.

Cardinal Godfried Danneels of Belgium, 2003

Abstinence before marriage and faithfulness to a single partner within a stable marriage—obviously, those are key to good living [and] to avoid infection. However, the church ministers in the real world. Not everybody follows the value-based calls that go out from the church. In that scenario, the church should give people [all] the options, one of which is to use a condom, not as a contraceptive, but to prevent transmission of a death-dealing virus.

Bishop Kevin Dowling of South Africa, 2004

The really sad thing is that none of these fundamentalist beliefs are grounded on, or representative of, the mainstream religions they profess to serve. Fundamentalist Christianity is widely considered as irrelevant to modern theology as it is to modern science. The extremist views and acts of fundamentalist Islam find little sanction in the Koran. . . . The campaign against the use of condoms is motivated by dogma, because it provides another example where faith and belief not only override evidence, but also lead to deliberate misrepresentation of the facts presumably in the service of a higher good. In this sense, it is a companion both in spirit and in tactical detail to the campaigns denying the reality of climate change or the seriousness of diminishing biodiversity.

Lord Robert May, president of the Royal Society, 2005

The danger is if we have a sort of blanket ban coming from the religious hierarchy saying it's wrong to do it, then you discourage people from doing it in circumstances where they need to protect their own lives. We are spending £1.5 billion over the next few years, trying to fight AIDS. It is also very important that we work on prevention and we are planning to uplift the amount of condoms that we will be distributing, too.

British prime minister Tony Blair, 2006

index